<u>Immunity Builders</u>

<u>Dedication</u>

I want to dedicate this book to my loving husband Apostle Stephen Spencer, all of my children Stephen, Alaysia, Joshua, Mariah, Josiah, and all of my grandchildren all of whom has stood by me and was a part of my journey and story. I give thanks to the Reformation Fellowship Tribe. I want to thank all of my followers on my live, Mother's Page, who has been so faithful and loyal. And last but not least I want to give a special thanks to Yolanda Griffin, for without her this book would have not been possible.

<u>Forward</u>

Apostle Dennese Spencer is a godly woman who has a energizing and contagious spirit. Mrs. Dennese Spencer is not a doctor, but, she is a certified health minister and wellness coach. Her goal is to have you healthy in your spirit, mind and body. It's very important to her to inform others about the importance of eating right. Her expertise is in health, and ministry. Her ministry is definitely lead by the Holy Spirit. Apostle Spencer is a wonderful mentor as well as the First Lady of El'Shaddai Ministries in Columbia, South Carolina. Dennese Spencer has done her research to be able to give you the information provided. She is married to Apostle Stephen Spencer and have been married to him for forty years. Apostle Dennese Spencer, better known as "Mother" or "Fire Starter" to all of those who knows her, has a great anointing over her life and has an intimate relationship with our Lord and Savior, Jesus Christ. She loves the Lord and is extremely faithful to Him as well as her husband, family and the church. It is an extreme blessing to have this mighty woman of God as a part of our lives.

<u>Introduction</u>

Building up your immune system is absolutely important especially if you want to survive in this world today. Our bodies needs the right nutrients to function correctly.Your diet can affect you mentally and physically. You should eat for your health and not by your emotions. Eating can either be beneficial to your body, or it can absolutely destroy it causing you all kinds of health issues.

Did you know that eating the right foods can give you a sense of peace, joy, happiness, enlightenment, and longevity? Who doesn't want this to be a part of their lifestyle? If you don't eat right you can develop memory lose, have hot flashes and night sweats. Not eating right can cause you to become fatigued and your energy level will decrease drastically. You'll wonder why you're having headaches, and are anxious and irritable all of the time. And for those of you who are married, do you know that what and how you eat can also affect your sex drive? Depending on what you eat, will cause you to develop water retention in your body and swelling in your legs. If you're a woman, you can develop heavy bleeding during your menstruation and your breasts will become tender which can develop small lumps that may lead to cancer. Your thinking can become foggy and you'll have what is called brain fog. This can happen in both men and women. You will have food cravings but for the wrong types of food. You can develop acne and just feel completely burned out. And this can happen to anyone. Women, you may have vaginal dryness and men, you can develop lower belly fat, develop erectile dysfunction and have an increase in urination. Both men and women will have a decrease in mental clarity, a decrease in your strength, poor blood concentration, and stiffness in your bones and body. You'll get offended easily making you to become very sensitive because food affects you emotionally as well.

Unknown to most people, words can also affect our health. Speaking and thinking positive things into and over your life, can uplift your spirit, your mood, and the people around you in a tremendous and remarkable way. Be mindful what you speak over yourself and others. Life and death is in the power of the tongue. Always do research on anything that you put in your body. Get into the habit of reading ingredients and the nutritional value of anything you purchase.

Table Of Content

Vegetables

Chapter One

Fruits

Fruits are natural sweeteners. Many people may not know that fruits boosts the immune system and have many benefits. They have many vitamins and are very healthy giving great benefits to your body.

Disclaimer:

There are fruits that are high in sugar and fruits that are low in sugar. Consult your doctor to see what fruits are good for your consumption especially if you're diabetic.

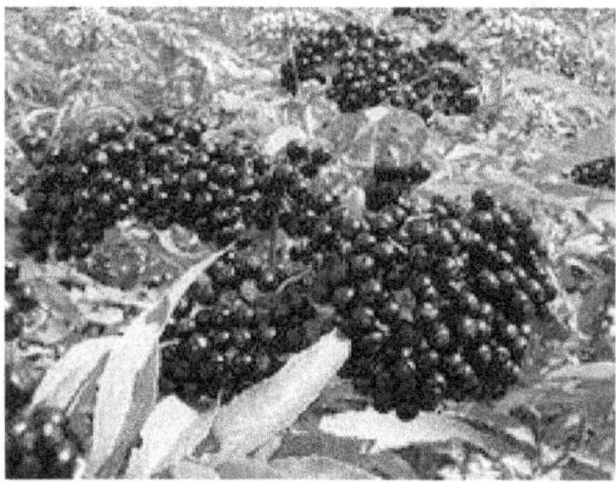

Elderberries

Elderberries can prevent cancer. They help with constipation and are an antidepressant. They are great for your well being and your emotions. They help with your digestion. They're great for cough, flues, cold, and viruses, such as the Corona Virus. They're good for sore throat, bone health and your bone tissue. You can add elderberries to your salad, in yogurt, or in a smoothie. Elderberries are high in sugar.

Smoothie

1 cup of Elderberries (fresh or frozen)
1 1/2 cup of unsweetened Almond milk
1 cup Spinach
1 frozen banana
1/2 cup of yogurt
Cinnamon (optional)

Fruit Bowl

1 1/2 cup yogurt	**Strawberries**
Elderberries	**Blackberries**
Banana	**Banana**
Honey	**Peaches**
Cinnamon	
Chia seeds	

Mix all ingredients in a bowl and enjoy

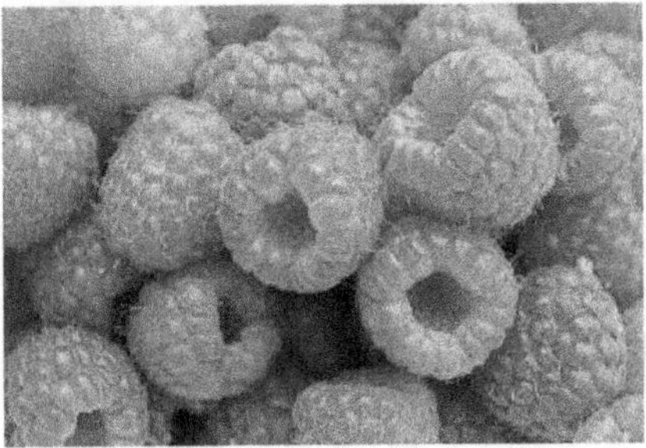

Raspberries

Raspberries have the vitamin B complex. They have vitamins K, C, and A. They are great for your heart health, and your digestion. Raspberries helps with inflammatory. You can add raspberries to your salad, put them into a smoothie or fruit bowl. Raspberries are low in sugar.

Smoothie

1 cup raspberries frozen or fresh
1 1/2 cup unsweetened almond milk, water
1 banana fresh or frozen
1/2 cup yogurt
1 Table spoon honey
1/2 cup ice
1 cup kale greens

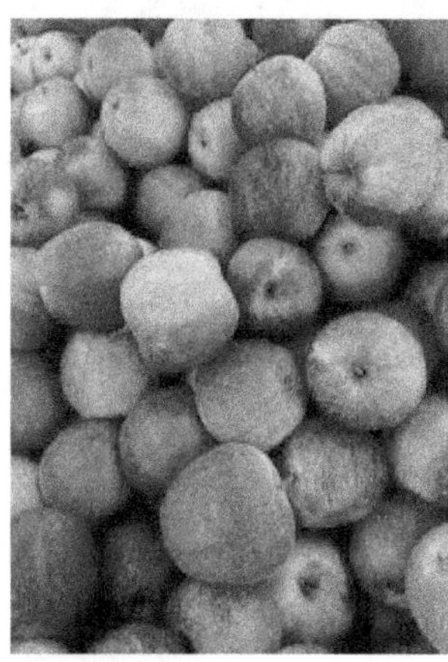

Apples help with dementia, cancer, the respiratory system, and the nervous system. They have iron, calcium, magnesium, and zinc. They also have vitamins A, C, E, K, and B. Apples can be added to salads or put into a smoothie. You can also put apples in your oatmeal for some added sweetness. Apples are low in sugar.

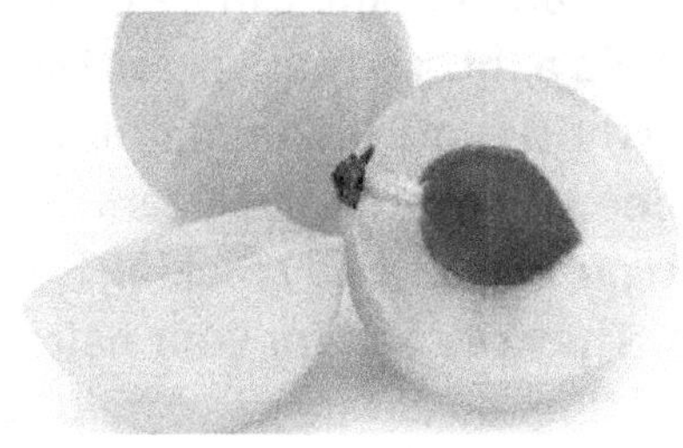

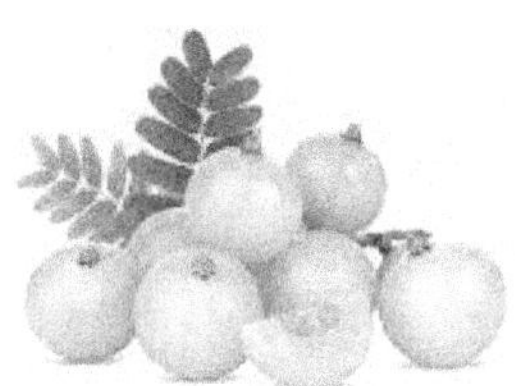

Amla Fruit are good for cough, your eyes, skin, hair, and you scalp. They do wonders for your nails and teeth. Alma Fruit helps with weight loss and anemia. It helps with concentration and intelligence. How great is that?! Have diarrhea, eat some Alma Fruit. It reduces swelling, and is great for your joints and arthritis. They help with your blood pressure and your nervous system. It help to fight bacteria and detoxifies the body. Alma fruit can help to increase your lifespan. They are wonderful for your vitality. It's an anti fungal, and is great for energy. Alma fruit are low in sugar.

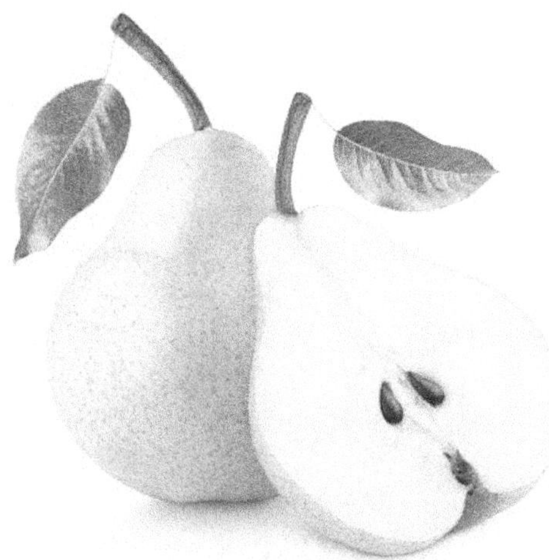

Pears have vitamin C which makes them good for coughs, colds, the flu, and viruses. Pears help to lower your blood pressure and helps with weight loss. Now who wouldn't want to lose some weight. Pears regulates your bowels and can help to prevent cancer. If you have a fever eating a pear will help a lot. They are great for your bone health which makes them good for, gout, arthritis, and inflammation. They help with swelling and mood swings. Have you been moody lately? Pears balances out your hormones. It regulates the blood sugar in your body making it great for diabetics. Pears prevent shortness of breath. They're good for your hair, skin, eyes, and helps treat wounds. They're also full of fiber so eat pears to help to keep you regular. Pears are low in sugar.

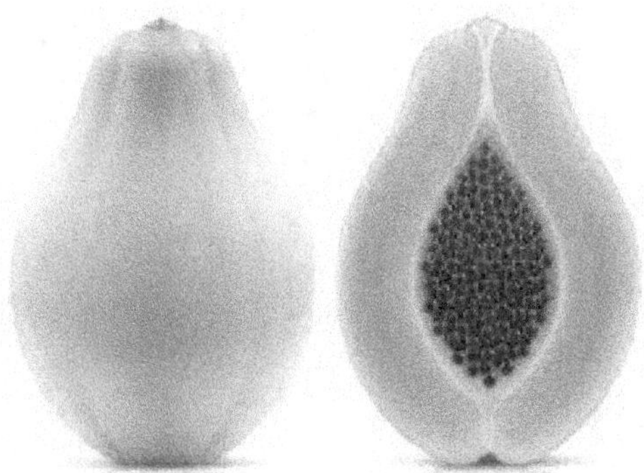

Papaya fruit kills viruses. Eating papaya helps to break down your food. They are good for your heart, and liver. Do you know papaya can help with acne and is good for your skin? Papaya helps with your menstrual cycle, nails, and your hair. Papaya does wonders for your body. They're great for your stomach, and your eyes. It lowers sugar levels making it great for diabetes. It helps with muscle degeneration, is good for your kidneys, and they have vitamin A. Papaya are low in sugar. Add papaya to a smoothie or a fruit bowl.

Smoothie

1 cup almond milk
1/4 cup Plain Greek yogurt
1 tsp pure vanilla extract
1 small ripe banana, peeled and sliced
1/2 large ripe papaya, peeled, seeded and cut into cubes
1 cup of ice (optional)

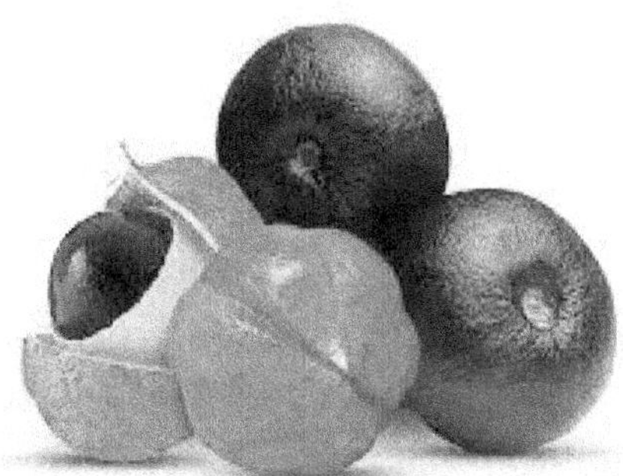

Gurana Fruit

Guarana Fruit helps to give your brain power. It helps you to focus, and concentrate. It helps to improve your memory, and increases your attention span. Your perception can become enhanced and it will helps you to perform tasks easily. Gurana helps to improve your sex drive, oh boy. It's great for your heart, and skin. It helps with fatigue, and it kills cancer cells. Gurana fruit helps with weight loss, is good for your kidneys and your blood flow. Gurana fruit is not a good choice to eat if you have diabetes.

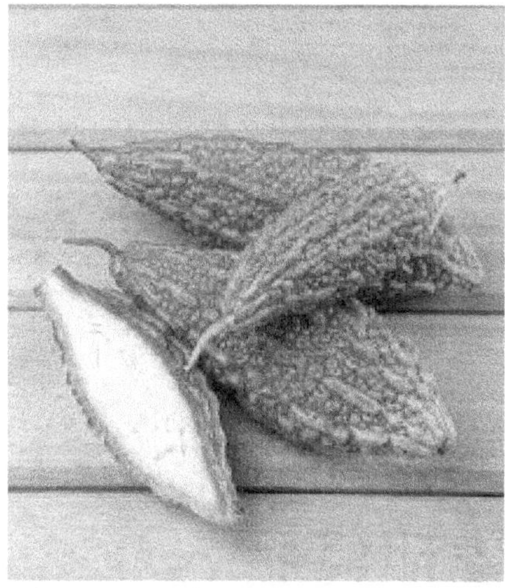

Bitter Gourd

Bitter Gourd detoxifies your body and helps to cleanse your blood and circulation. It's good for energy, stamina, gout, and arthritis. Your eyesight will improve. It's great for the respiratory system, your liver, and skin. It kills parasites, and kill germs. It's an antibiotic, and an antiseptic. Bitter gourd is low in sugar.

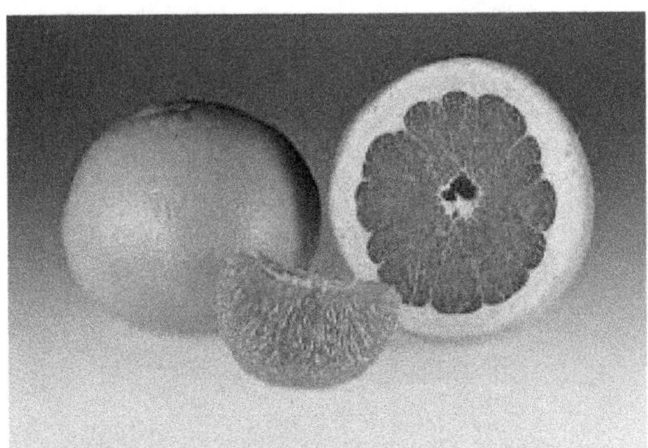

Grapefruit has vitamins C, B, D, E, and K. It has potassium, and electrolytes. It alkaline the body, and helps to fight cancer. Grapefruit kills bacteria, and renews your tissues. It's good for swelling, and inflammation. It helps with asthma, your digestive system, your heart, and fights fungus. Grapefruit is low in sugar.

Fruit Bowl

Yogurt (Plain Greek Yogurt)
1/2 Grapefruit
Honey
Strawberries
Banana
Granola
Cinnamon
Flax Seeds
Blueberries
Grapes

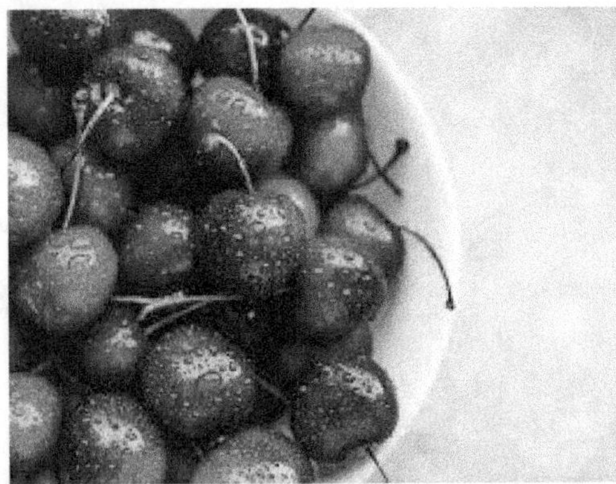

Cherries are good for bone health making them great for arthritis and gout. They're good for your blood circulation, your muscles, brain function, and Dementia. If you're constipated cherries would be a great laxative. Cherries helps with Parkinson Disease. Cherries are great for your liver, your kidneys, mood swings, and depression. They help to fight cancer and to prevent strokes. Cherries are good for anti-aging and they're anti-inflammatory. They help to promote good sleep giving you peaceful rest. It helps with your sex life especially for married couples. It has magnesium, melatonin, and vitamin C making it great for colds, the flu, and viruses. Cherries helps with constipation and your urine. Cherries are high in sugar.

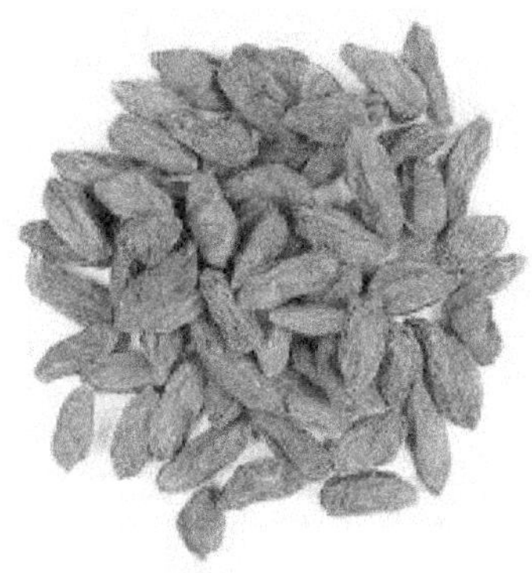

Goji Berry

Goji Berry is good for cough, colds, and the flu. It has vitamins E, A, B12, and C. It helps to prevent liver infection. Goji Berries is a fat burner. They help to prevent cancer, anxiety, stress, depression, and dry coughs. They help to regulate your blood sugar making it great for diabetics. It's good for gut health, energy, and your well being. Women, Goji Berries are good if you're going through menopause. And they are good for your vision, nerves, and your kidneys. Goji berries are low in sugar.

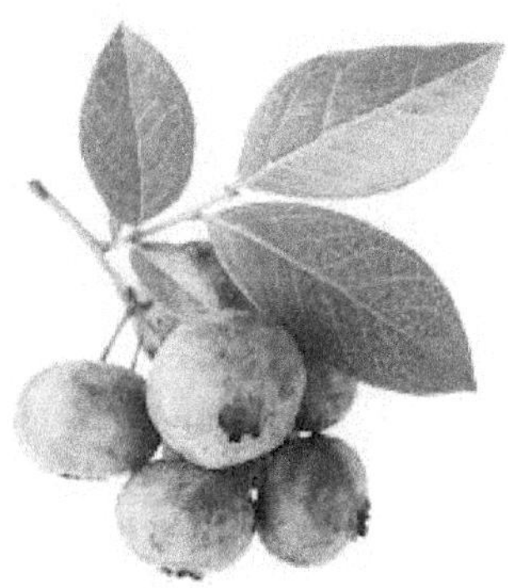

Bilberry Fruit

Bilberry fruit has vitamins A, B, C, zinc, and iron. It helps the brain to function well making it good for your memory, it gives your clarity. They lower your blood pressure and helps with Dementia. They help with forgetfulness. Eating Bilberry fruit helps with bruising and are great for your eyes, helping to prevent glaucoma. It helps to regulate your blood sugar making it great for diabetics. Its good for kidneys infection and kidney damage. They help to prevent blood clots. Bilberries soothes throat irritation and fatigue so eat some to boost your energy. They help with arthritis, gout, and your bones. They also help to prevent breast cancer, colon cancer, and Leukemia. Bilberries are low in sugar.

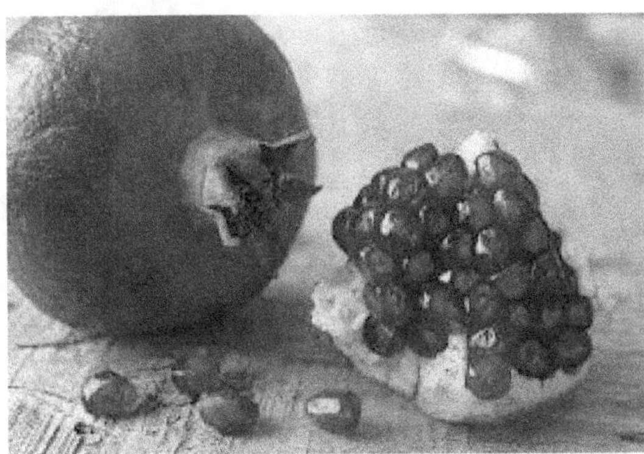

Pomegranate

Pomegranate has vitamins , D, B6, and iron. Pomegranate helps to fight breast cancer, prostate cancer, and lung cancer. They it help support prostate health, and it helps with erectile dysfunction. Eating pomegranate helps to lower your blood pressure. They're great for joint pain, arthritis, and gout. They help with fever, your bones, and your arteries. Want stamina, eat some pomegranate. They are good for your brain, making them great for Dementia. They help to clean your arteries, and does wonders for your skin, hair, nails and PMS. It lowers your cholesterol level and helps to rid the body of intestinal worms and parasites. Pomegranate are low in sugar.

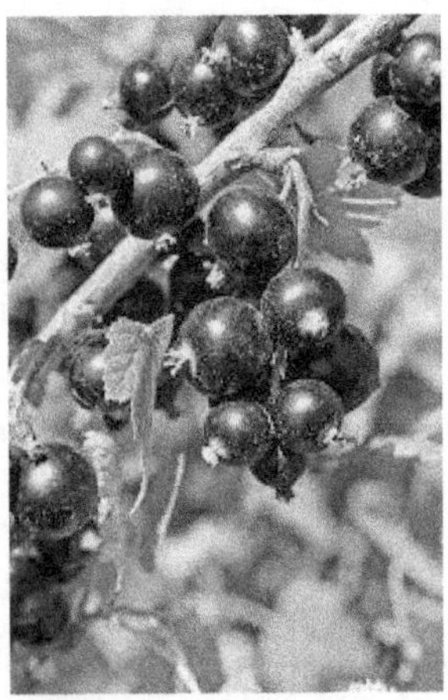

Black Currant

Black Currant it has vitamins C, B5, B6, B1, E zinc, iron, calcium, folate, and magnesium. It helps with mood swings, and memory loss making it great for Alzheimer's Disease making it good for your brain. Black currant helps with your blood flow, sore throat, your hair, nails, and and skin. I helps to prevent premenstrual syndrome. Black currant are low in sugar.

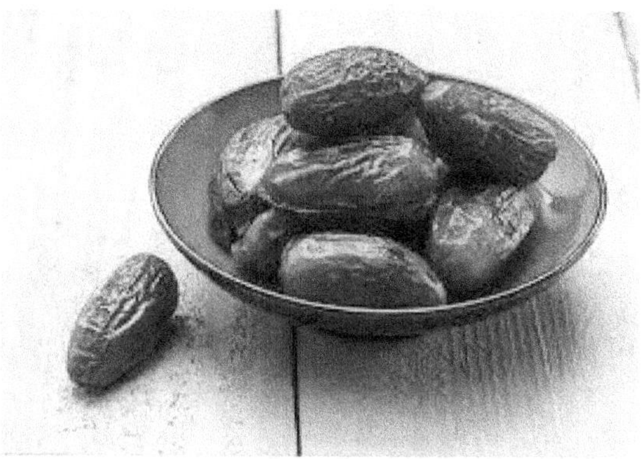

Dates

Dates are great for your hormones, bones, gout, bone pain, and arthritis. Dates will help with constipation, your skin, and your eyes. It helps with your digestive system and helps with diarrhea. Eating dates lowers your blood pressure and gives your energy. They are good for your memory, and helps to give you clarity. They also help with Alzheimer and Dementia. Dates has vitamins B1, B2, B3, B5, magnesium, folate acid, and potassium. They help to prevent heart attacks and sexual weakness. Dates are low in sugar.

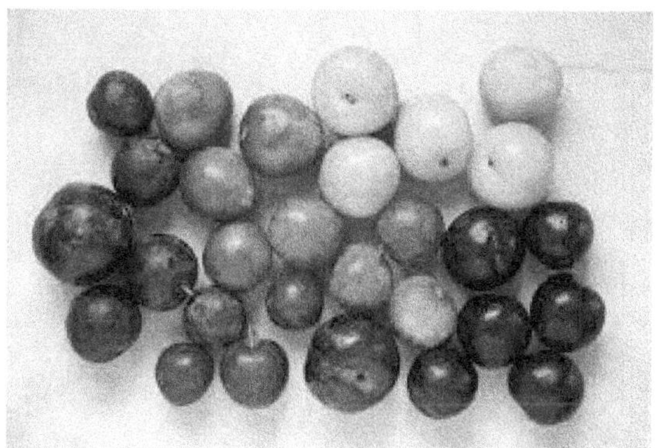

Plums

Plums increases your memory, your concentration, and your intelligence. Plums detoxes the body, and gives you energy. Plums are good for your bones, arthritis, and gout. They're good for your blood and helps to fight cancer. They are good in preventing stomach worms. Plums are good for your heart, tonsils, gums, and your skin. It's great if your anemic, and helps with weight loss so eat some plums. Plum are great for, coughs, colds, the flu, and viruses. They have vitamins E, K and zinc. They are also an anti-aging fruit, and great for pregnant women. Plums are low in sugar.

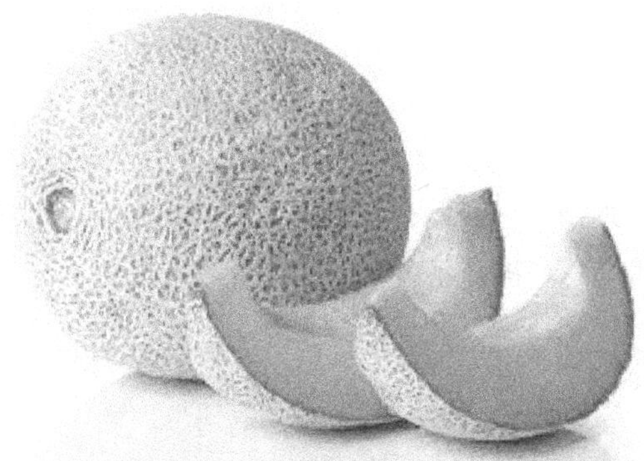

<u>Cantaloupe</u>

Cantaloupes has vitamins B6, B9 and C. It's good for colds, the flu, cough. They help to prevent leg cramps, arthritis, gout, and your bones. They are low in sugar and are high in fiber. Cantaloupe reduces water retention in your body. It promotes lung health and prevents heart disease. They reduce your blood pressure and is good for your hair, skin, and your intelligence. Cantaloupes prevents wrinkles, prevents urinary tract infections, and helps to prevents cancer. They reduce kidney dysfunction, constipation, gas and helps with fever. Cantaloupes also helps with arthritis, gout and your bones. Cantaloupe are low in sugar.

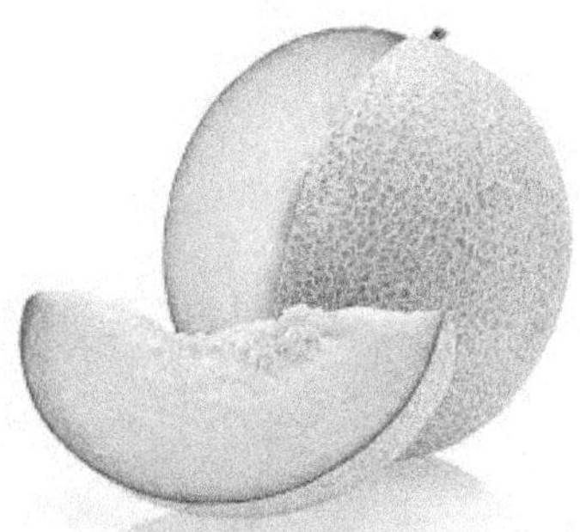

<u>Honey Dew Melon</u>

Honey dew has the vitamin B complex, E, C, A, potassium, iron, and magnesium. It's full of fiber helping to regulate your bowels. It helps with colds, the flu, and cough. It's wonderful if you have a child with ADHD, or an adult with ADDHD. Honey dew melons.They lower the risk of heart attacks and strokes. It's helps to speed up wound healing. Honey dew regulates your blood sugar, which is especially good for diabetes. They help to keep your skin from sagging. Don't you want to eat more of this fruit ?! It regulates your blood pressure, and strengthens your bones and teeth. Eating honey dew melons helps to hydrate your body. It help with is stress, can you imagine that? it prevents eye disease,and can improve your body performance. Honey dew enhances your mood and improves your memory. Wow, what a great fruit. Honey dew melon are low in sugar.

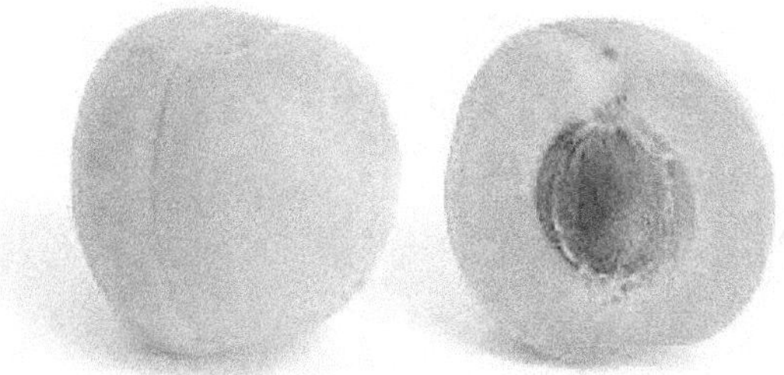

Apricots helps with colds, coughs, the flu and viruses. it has vitamins C, A, iron, potassium, and copper. The seed has vitamin B17, you can add the seed to your smoothie. Apricots are a natural laxative because it contains fiber. It helps to a prevent fatty liver. It does wonders for an earache and fever. They also balance the electrolyte in your body. Apricots are low in sugar.

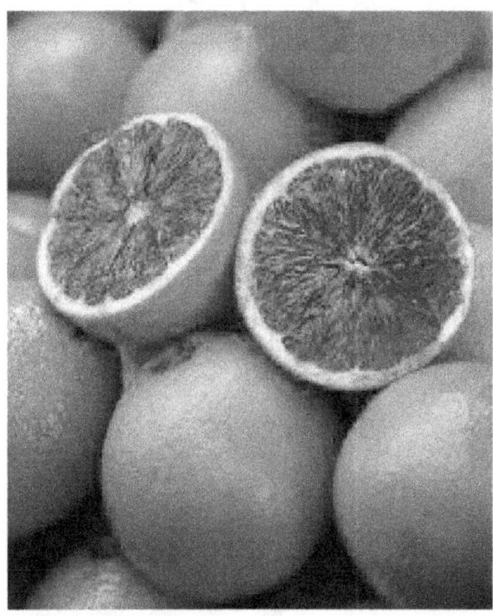

Blood orange are full of vitamins and minerals. They have vitamins A the B complex, and folate. It helps with colds, cough, the flu and viruses. It lowers your blood pressure,and helps with inflammation. They help to prevent pain and swelling in your body. Blood orange helps to prevent muscle spasms, fights against cancer, and prevents toxins from building up in your body. They stimulate your liver and is good for you if you are anemic, because they build up and aid with the growth of red blood cells. They are great for your emotions by alleviating stress and depression. They are good in fighting infections and help with healing wounds. They fight germs, are good for your eyes, teeth and bones. Blood orange improves your blood circulation, and helps with fetal development. They help with your digestion, vital organs, and they protect your skin. They also help with the development of collagen, and weight control. They and are good for your hormones, gives you energy, and supports the functions of your kidneys, along with filtering out the toxins in your kidneys. Blood orange are high in sugar.

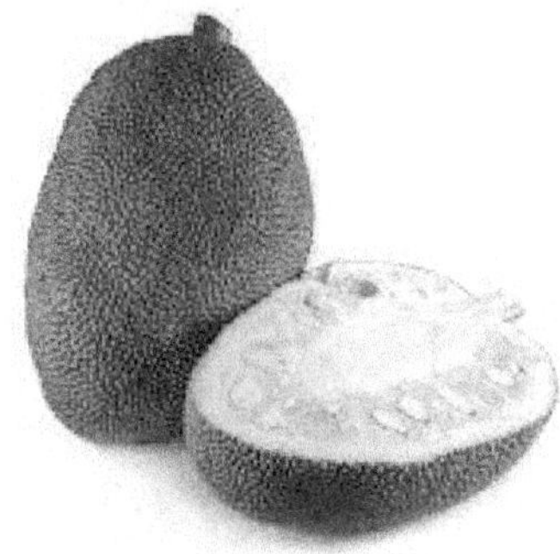

Jackfruit has vitamins B12, B1, C, A, magnesium, calcium, and Omega 3. It's good for colds, coughs and the flu,.It advances the oxygen in your body and helps with the circulation of your blood. It boosts your energy, lowers your blood pressure, and regulates your blood sugar making it great for diabetics. Jackfruit helps to prevent all forms of cancer. They strengthens your bones, and helps to prevent gout and joint pain. It helps with fractures, constipation and fever. It's good for your skin is anti-aging, now who doesn't want to look younger? Jackfruit are low in sugar.

Chapter 2

Fluids
Unknown to most, many teas helps to boost the immune system and offers many benefits, so grab a cup of tea and enjoy knowing that you are getting great taste and great health benefits.

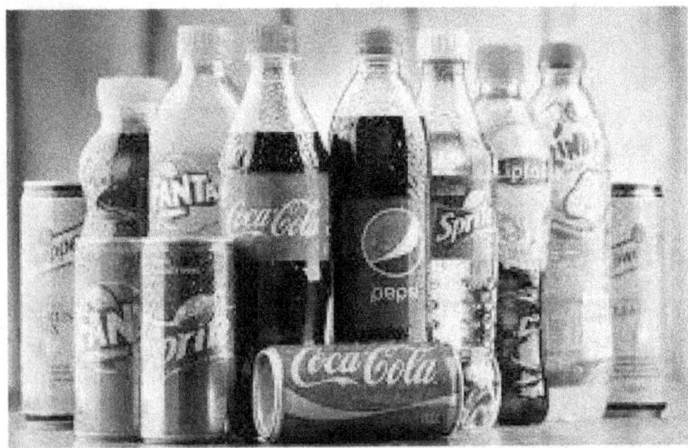

Soda

Do Not Drink Soda!!! Soda causes headaches, dizziness, anxiety, aggression, and seizures. Soda erodes your teeth and bones. They increase the effect of asthma attacks. Soda can promote breast cancer and men will have a higher risk of heart attacks, and soda your disrupts hormones. Soda promotes brain cancer and causes toxic to the brain. It hardens your arteries and causes weight gain. Are you wondering why you may not be losing weight, maybe it's because you're drinking soda. It cause rashes and damages your nerves. One soda per day increases the risk of diabetes and diet sodas are the worst to drink. Stay Away From The Soda!!

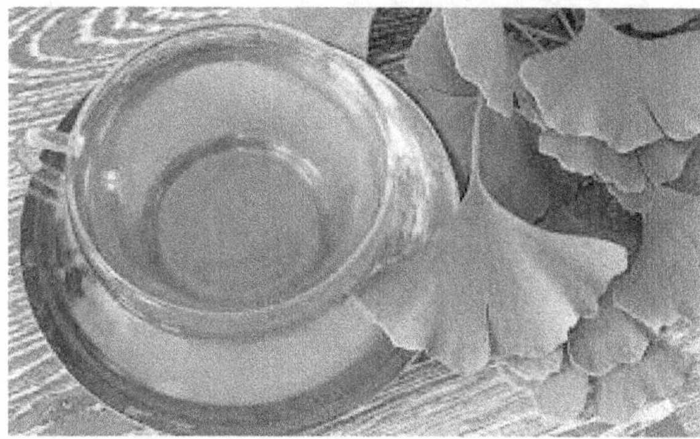

Ginkgo tea enhances energy and motivation. It improves your blood circulation, and improves and increases dilation of your blood vessels. It shields and strengthens your heart. It enhances the dopamine levels in your body and regulate high blood pressure. Its anti-aging, helps with your memory, and reduces migraine headache. It helps you to focus more and lengthens your attention span. Ginkgo tea helps you to overcome depression, prevents cancer, and reduces the risk of nervous disorders. It helps with memory loss, making it extremely helpful for Alzheimer and Dementia. It helps with ringing in the ears, reduces DNA damage, and improves your ability to learn new tasks.

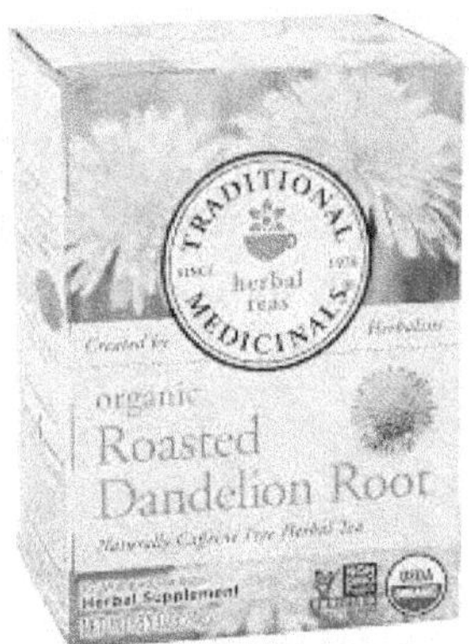

Dandelion tea stimulates the neurons in your brain. It deletes low self-esteem and removes toxins out of your body. Dandelion tea puts oxygen in your body, and resets and repairs your gut and liver. It speeds up weight loss, and cleanses your blood tissues. It helps your organs and glands and, increases your energy. It also gets rid of things in your body.

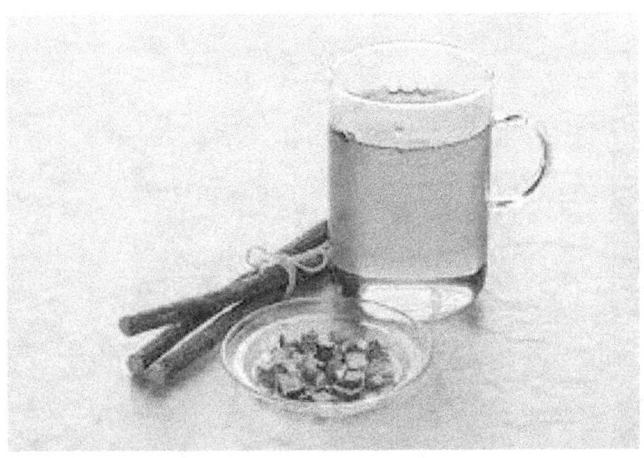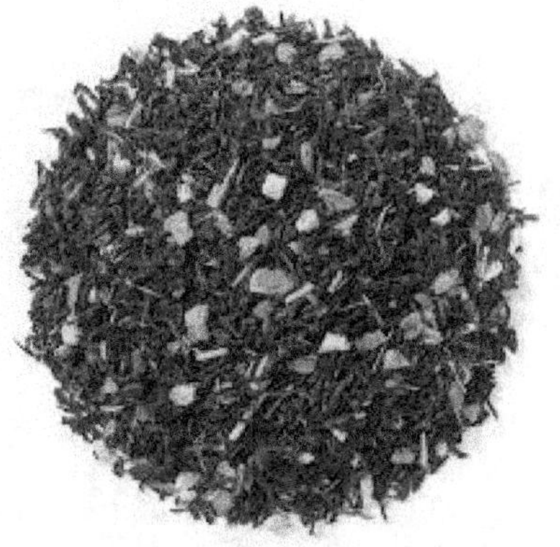

Licorice tea is good for your eyes, lungs, and anxiety. It helps with mood swings, cancer, and depression. It's good for your lungs and is great for you if you have herpes. It's good for diabetics, and helps your brain and your mentality.

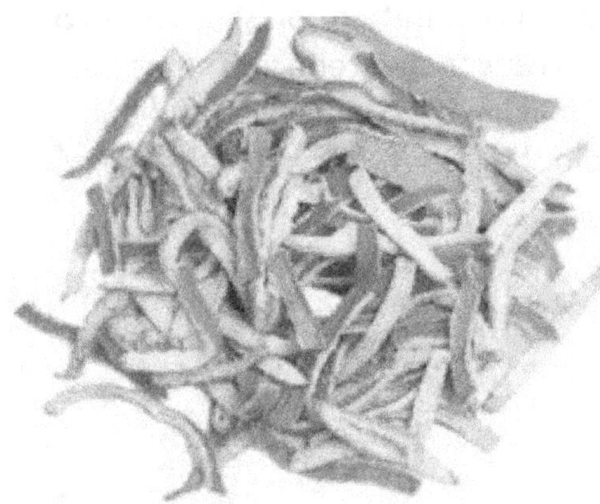

Orange peel has vitamin C, and is good for colds, coughs, and the flu. It's good for your hair, nails, skin, and acne. Orange peel tea if great for your digestive system and your heart. It helps to fight cancer and fights inflammation. It fights against swelling, bloating and is good for your bowels.

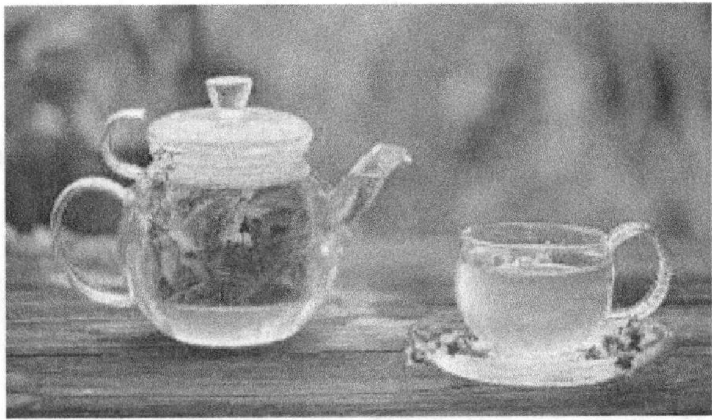

You can get Green tea in powder form. Green tea is good for your eyes, blood cells, brain cells,and your teeth and gums. Green tea helps to fight cavities, and is good if you have asthma. It's good for the cold, the flu, and helps to fight viruses. If you have arthritis and inflammation this tea will be good for you. It helps with your memory and Dementia. It helps to burns fat and is good helps for your blood circulation. Do you know that green tea can unclog your pores? It slows down the aging process. It reduces plaque and helps to remove kidney stones. Green tea assists in weight loss, stress and depression. It's also great and is for lowering your blood pressure.

Green tea fights bladder infection, changes your mood, and fights cancer cells. It helps you to relax. This tea is good for your bones, helps to heal wounds, and is good for asthma. Green tea fights bacteria and, it's good for your skin. It gives you energy, and is good if you're anemic. it has vitamins B, iron, and magnesium. This tea also helps with inflammation. It's such a beneficial tea.

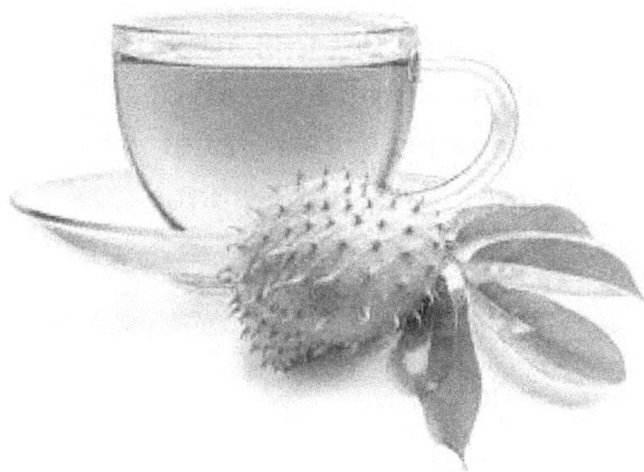

Soursop Tea

Soursop tea helps to regulate your blood pressure, and is anti-inflammatory. It's high in antioxidants, has antibacterial benefits, and can help to fight cancer.

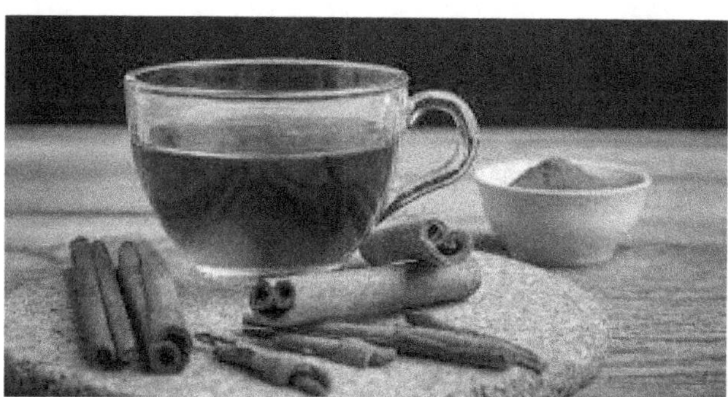

Cinnamon Tea

Cinnamon tea fights viruses, colds, the flu and a sore throat. It fights stomach pain, cramps, and acid reflux. It helps if you have high blood pressure and it fights bacteria.

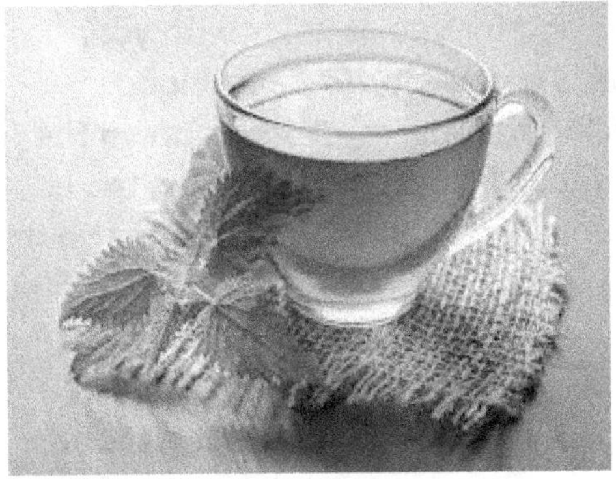

Peppermint tea is a good to drink and is a good air freshener, just put some in a pot on the stove and enjoy the smell. It's good for coughs, colds, the flu, viruses, and allergies. It helps with cantor sores and is good to help stop vomiting. Want your hair to grow? Well, this tea is great for that. Peppermint tea helps to relive cramps and mosquito bites. It does wonders for your skin by fighting acne. Having problems with diarrhea? Here's a good remedy. This tea is good for your brain, and is good to drink for pregnant woman experiencing morning sickness. It helps to keep you alert and is good for your bones. It has vitamins C, B, potassium magnesium and calcium.

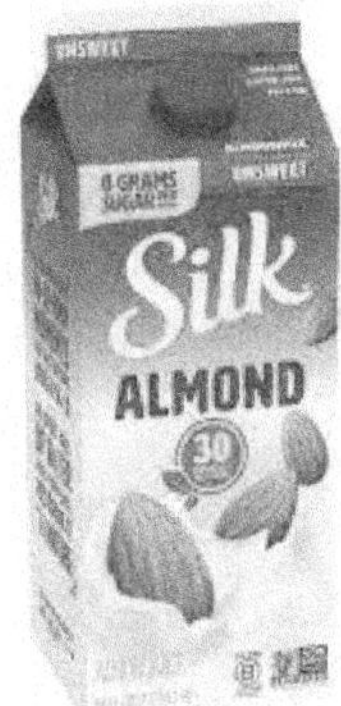

Guess what? Almond milk is better to drink than regular milk. It builds up your immune system and helps to prevent cancer. Almond milk helps to repair damaged skin and reduces the risk of heart disease, It helps to regulate your blood pressure and it reduces the risk of arthritis. It also gives you good healthy kidneys and improves your vision. This is such a great milk alternative.

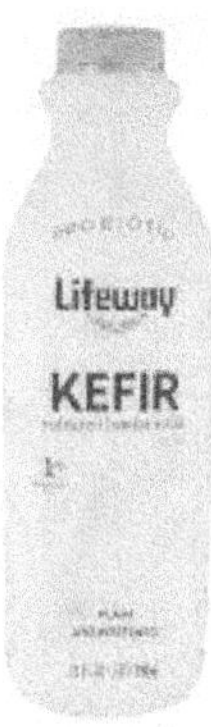

<u>Kefir</u>

Kefir is good for your gut health. It's another alternative to milk. It helps with urinary tract infections. It helps with ulcer, and helps with diarrhea. It reduces your appetite making it a helpful choice for weight loss. it regulates your blood sugar which is great for diabetics. Kefir helps to reduce tumors, wow, imagine that! And Kefir is good for the health of your bones. It is a pro-biotic and is good for your brain. Kefir is also an antibiotic.

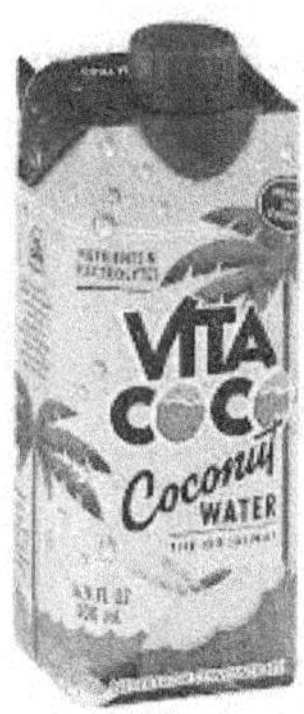

<u>Cocont Water</u>

Coconut water is good for your skin, hair growth, and hair breakage. Coconut water helps with weight loss and it helps you to concentrate more, oh we all need that. It helps with your memory which is good for Dementia and Alzheimer's. It's good for your heart and your digestion. Coconut water helps to relive muscle cramps and it helps to flush your kidneys. You can drink this to get rid of worms and parasites, and we all have parasites, some of us has more than others. It has vitamins and minerals such as vitamins C, calcium and magnesium. It helps with depression and anxiety. It's good to prevent bloating as well. It gives you strength, is good for diabetics and helps with your blood circulation.

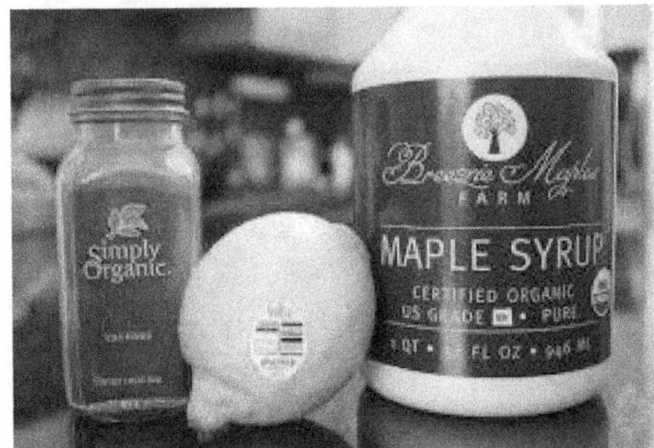

Lemonade Cleanser

A lemonade cleanser is great for your body. It contains lemons of cause or 100 percent lemon juice, apple cider vinegar, cayenne pepper, water, honey and cinnamon. Its full of vitamins and minerals. It is good for diabetics by regulating your blood sugar. it reduces your blood pressure, helps to clear your sinuses, and is good for good blood circulation. This is a very healthy drink and very beneficial to drink especially, if you are fasting. It's best to drink this on an empty stomach and drinking it warm or at room temperature.

Your body will let you know when it needs to be cleansed. It will let you know if you become constipated. It will help if you're bloated or you have gas. If your stomach protrudes, or you are in a lot of pain, drink a cup of lemonade cleanser. This drink can help if you have unexpected weight gain. It helps if you have intense food cravings. It's beneficial if you are moody, depressed, sluggish, or fatigued. Drink some of this if you have problems sleeping, have a headache, or have worms. Cleansing your body will flatten your stomach and increase your confidence and can give you courage.

Ingredients For Lemonade Cleanse

10 fluid oz purified water
2 Tbs lemon juice
2 Tbs maple syrup
1/8 tsp cayenne pepper
Stir ingredients until well mixed

Chapter 3
Beneficial Spices, Herbs, Powders, And Seasonings

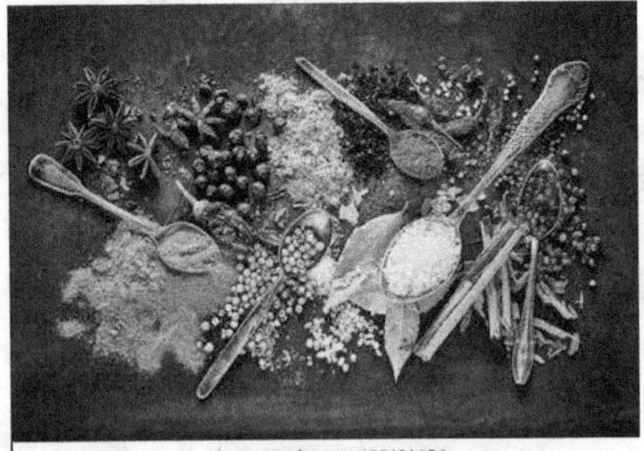

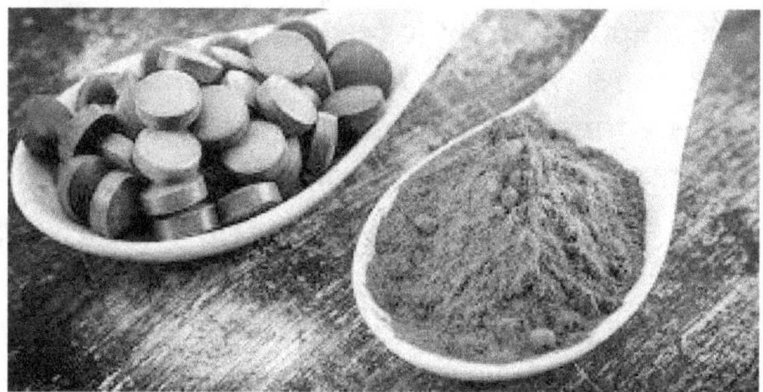

Chlorella has the B complex and and vitamin C. It detoxifies your blood, and removes bacteria and poison from your blood. It removes pollutants and mold from your body, yes, you can have mold in your body. It increases your stamina and your energy. Chlorella makes you feel good and enthusiastic. Its good for bone growth, and helps with ADD and ADDHD. It improves the symptoms of breast cancer, and it helps to prevent all cancers. It will help you to focus and concentrate. Chlorella strengthens the function of your liver. Taking Chlorella prevents the swelling of your joints. This is the highest known source for iron and protein. Its good for arthritis, and it fights infections. It aids with diabetes and fights fatigue. This is good for colds allergies, sores, nose congestion, brain infection and Alzheimer.

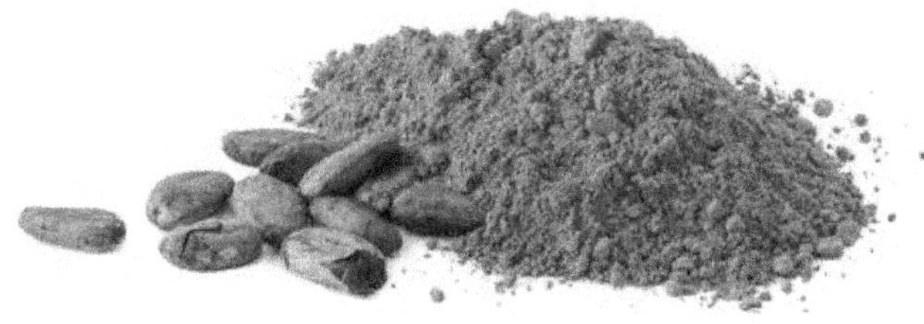

shutterstock.com · 766656388

Cocoa comes from a tree and is a good coffee substitute. It does have a bitter taste and was known as food of the gods. Cocoa reduces cataracts and reduces PMS symptoms. It's an antioxidant and it helps with the function of the brain. Cocoa can help to regulate your blood pressure and can help to reduce the risk of strokes and heart attacks. Its good for your bones, arthritis, and gout. Cocoa helps you to focus and to stay alert. Cocoa has omega 6, magnesium, folate acid, protein, and caffeine. Cocoa is a super food, and it helps if you're diabetic because it helps to regulate your blood sugar. It helps you to relax and it detoxes the body. This powder helps to fight cancer. It also helps with your bowels. Cocoa repairs your skin and can reduce cellulite. Cocoa firms your skin and manages depression. It helps to alleviate stress and enhances you physically. Cocoa is good for your nerves, your muscle function, and lifts your mood. It supports weight loss, gives you energy, and releases your happy hormones. And you know what else, it releases chemicals that gives you the feeling of bliss. It slows down the aging process and gives you stamina. Its great for you physically and mentally, but its not good for you if you have kidney problems.

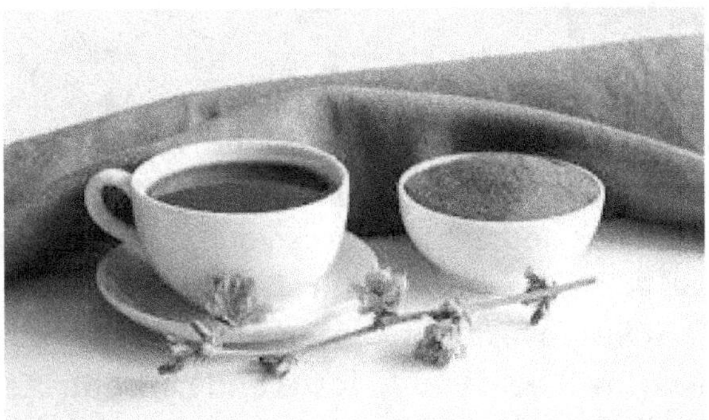

Chicory

Chicory has vitamins B12, B2, A, C and fiber. Chicory is good for colds, coughs and the flu. It relieves joint pain and heart pain. Chicory helps with heart disease, acid reflux, and heart burn. It prevents urinary tract disease and is great for your kidneys. It helps to fight bladder infection, anxiety, stress, and depression. Chicory will lower your blood pressure as well. It detoxes the spleen, and is a mild laxative. It enhances the calcium to absorb in your body. It reduces the ability of bone fractures which makes it good for your bone health. This is wonderful if you have gout, arthritis or joint pain. It reduce uric acid is good for your bowels especially if you're constipated. Its good for your hair, nails and skin.

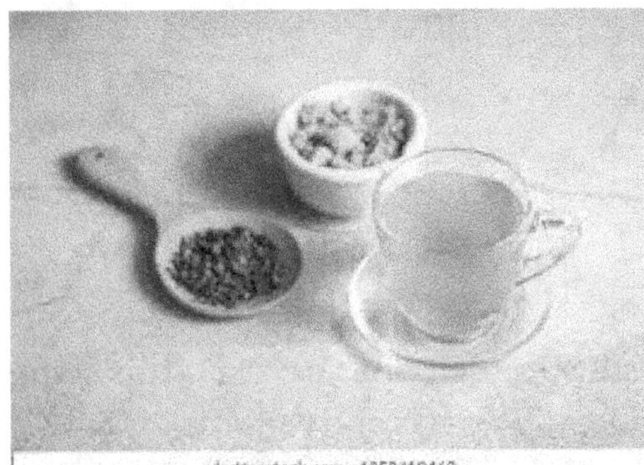

Yellow Cloves

Yellow cloves is good for your if you are experiencing any pain. It's great for your skin, bones, and your joints. Yellow cloves can help to stop a runny nose, and helps with muscle spasms. Using yellow cloves helps with bloating, vomiting, and your respiratory system. Having problems with arthritis? Use some in your food. It's help for coughs, the flu,and colds. It helps to relieve headaches, helps with swelling, and it fights against bacteria. Taking yellow cloves helps to regulate your blood sugar so it's good for diabetics. It helps to heal your body inside and out. It's also and antiseptic and air freshener. To freshen the air drop some in a pot on the stove, heat it up and enjoy the smell. It has vitamins K,B,E, and C, you can add it to your tea for a delightful boost in taste and it helps to prevent cancer.

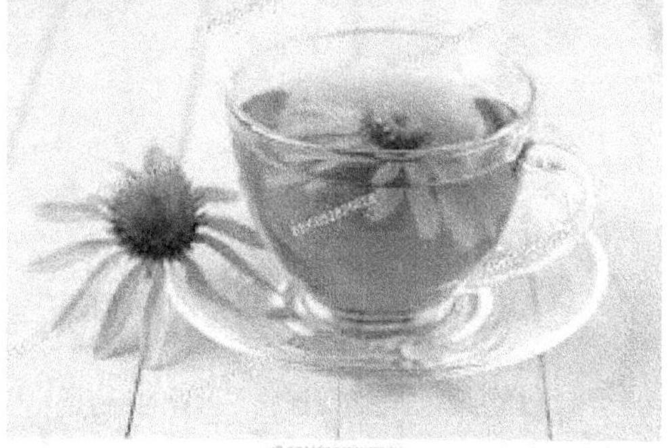

The Benefits Of Echinacea

Echinacea helps to fight against the Covid-19. Everyone should definitely use this. It lowers stress and helps to prevent heart attacks and heart disease. Echinacea helps to fight infections, repairs tissues, and help to prevent cancer. It does wonders for urinary tract infection. It lowers stress and swelling, and is great for your skin, hair, and nails. It helps to prevent diarrhea, and it fights bacteria. This is great for coughs, colds and the flu.

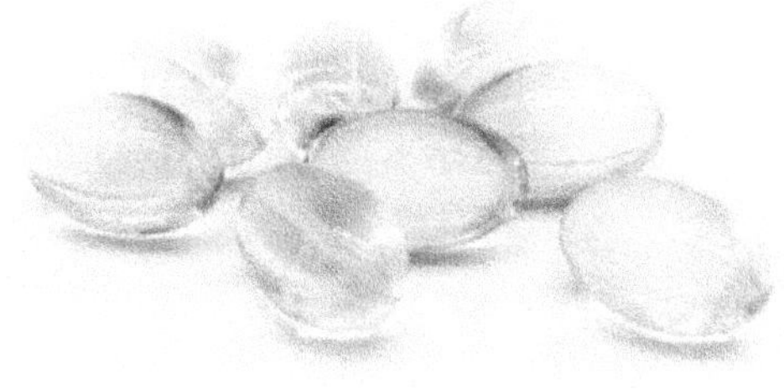

Omega- 3,6,9;

Omega 3-6-9 are great for you if you have a sore throat. This product is good for your skin, your eyes, and helps with the function of your brain. They support the nervous system and can prevent inflammation. Omega 3-6-9 helps to prevent learning disabilities.They also help with your blood circulation. You a can find Omega 3-6-9, in salmon, tuna, sardines, kale, walnuts, eggs, flax seeds, and chia seeds. They also have iron in it. They are great for arthritis, diabetics, helps to fight allergies. Are you going through menopause? Well I truly recommend this. It's great for your reproductive system, high blood pressure, hair growth and cancer. You can get Omega 3,6,9 in pill form and powder form as well.

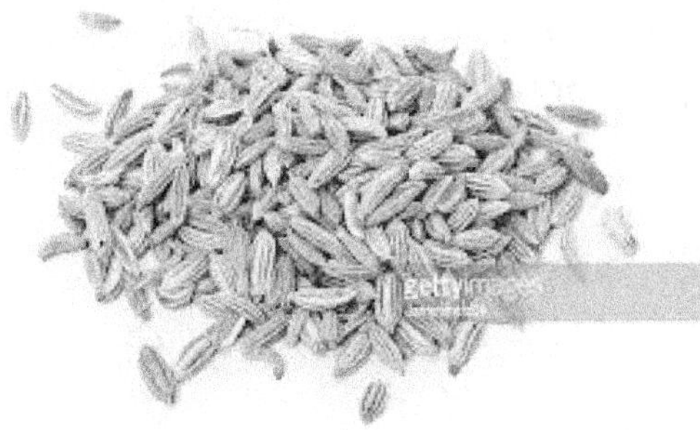

Fennel

Fennel is good for cough, cold, the flu and viruses. Did you know that Fennel is a medicine and a spice? It helps with weight loss, your heart, and your mental health. It can do wonders with those who has Alzheimer's disease. Going through menopause? Please add Fennel to your food. Fennel helps with androgynous, inflammation, swelling, and mood swings. It helps to prevent bloating and prevents water retention. This is great if you have arthritis. It help with the function of your brain. Fennel is good for your bones and your lungs. It helps with gas, your stomach, and your blood. Fennel has folate, potassium, magnesium, and vitamins C and B6, it also has calcium.

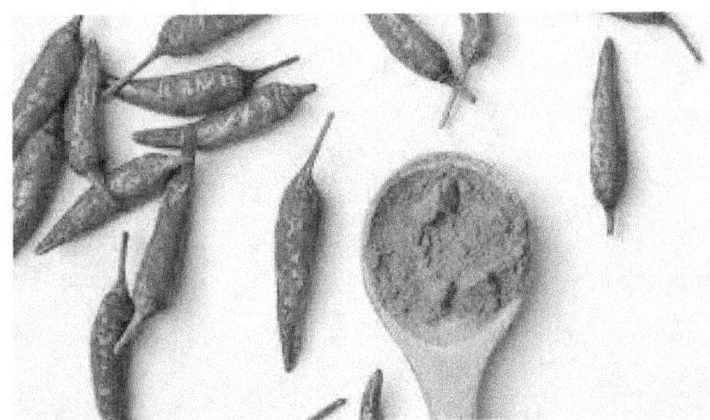

Cayenne Pepper

Cayenne pepper is a spice that helps with colds, coughs, the flu, and viruses. It has vitamins A, E and C. Cayenne pepper actually helps with memory loss, and your blood flow. It helps to prevent stomach ulcers and is great for your heart. If you have a headache add some cayenne pepper to some of your food. Adding cayenne pepper to your dishes can help if you have asthma. It does wonder for your intestines as well as your blood. This spice helps with shingles and arthritis. It helps to lower the blood sugar in your body, so it's great for diabetics. Do you have a cold an are congested adding this spice will help a great deal. It helps to detox the body and helps with your cholesterol.

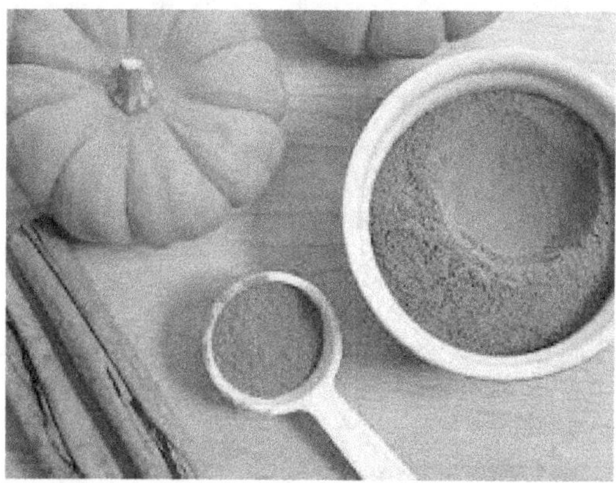

<u>Pumpkin Spice</u>

Pumpkin spice is good for your eyes, your heart, and your brain. This wonderful spice gives you a healthy liver and aids in your digestion. It helps to clear up a runny nose. It's great for diabetics by it regulating the insulin in your body. If you're having problems sleeping, this spice helps with your insomnia. It helps to remove mucus and is good for the flu,and viruses. It releases the serotonin in your body. Pumpkin spice has the B complex, magnesium, iron, and calcium and it also helps to fight cancer.

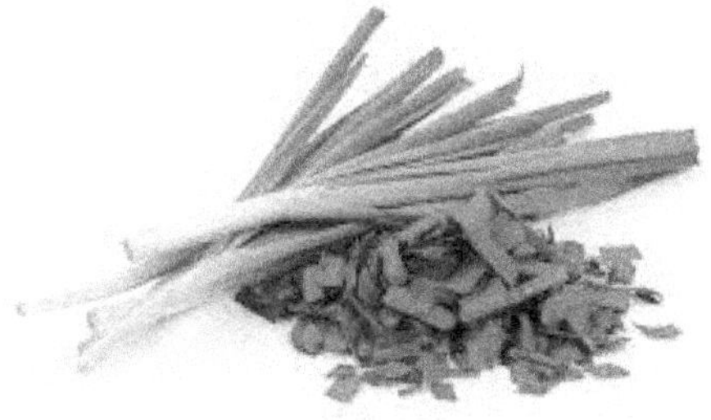

<u>Chives</u>

Chives are good for the flu, cough, cold, and viruses because it has vitamin C. It helps with your heart, unclogs your arteries and your blood vessels. Chives are great for arthritis, gout and bone density. It helps if you have any inflammation, swelling, or bruising. It has contains vitamins A, K, and C, zinc, magnesium, and calcium. It is a natural pain killer, and helps to calms you. It's good if you are anemic and helps to fight cancer. What a wonderful spice. It helps with your digestive system, and is great for pregnant women and babies. This spice actually detoxifies the body. It helps to expel mucus and is also good for your skin. It also helps your urinary tract.

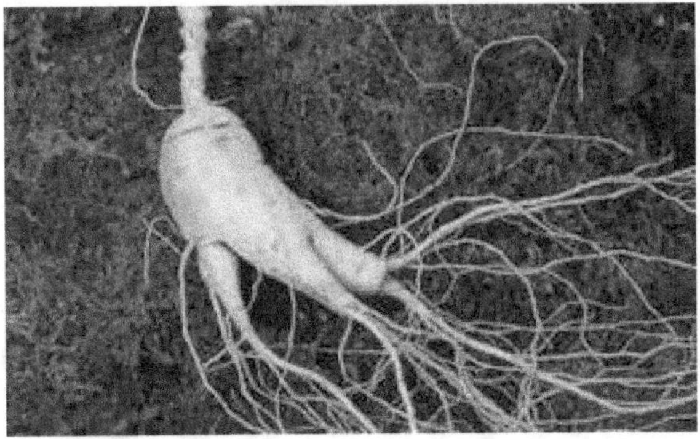

Indian Ginseng helps if you are having issues with your thyroids, but it's not good for you if you have high blood pressure, talk to your doctor first. It helps to fight off cancer cells and helps with Parkinson Disease, arthritis. Indian ginseng is great to take for your heart and helps if you are going through any depression. If you are having mood swings, this would be great to have on hand. This can build your confidence, and men, it increases your sperm count. It regulates your blood sugar making it great for diabetics, and helps people with Alzheimer Disease so if you have a loved on suffering with this please incorporate Indian Ginseng in their diet. Indian Ginseng is great for your well being as a whole. You can get this in pill, powder or tea form.

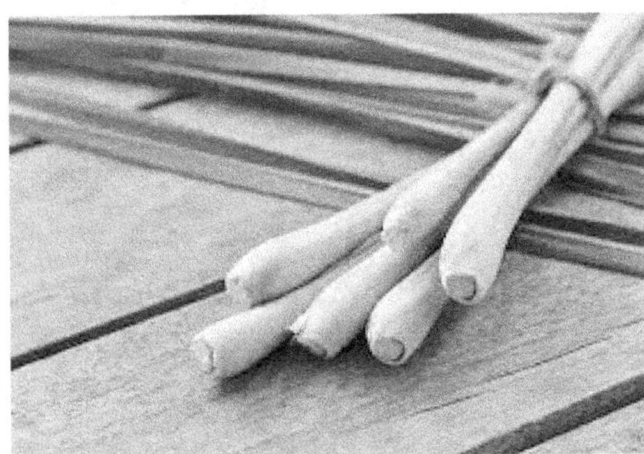

Lemongrass fights infections, it helps with lowering a fever. Add Lemongrass to your diet to help to fight depression, and mood swings. It helps to regulate your blood pressure, is good for your nervous system. If you're having issues with your stomach eat Lemongrass. Lemongrass is good for your bladder, your kidneys, your liver, and your urinary tract. It's good for gout, your bones, and arthritis. It's good to eat for colds, coughs, and the flu because It contains vitamin C. It also helps to prevent aches and pains.

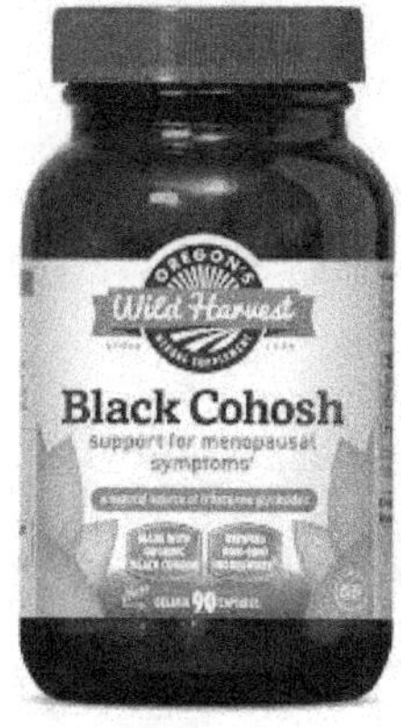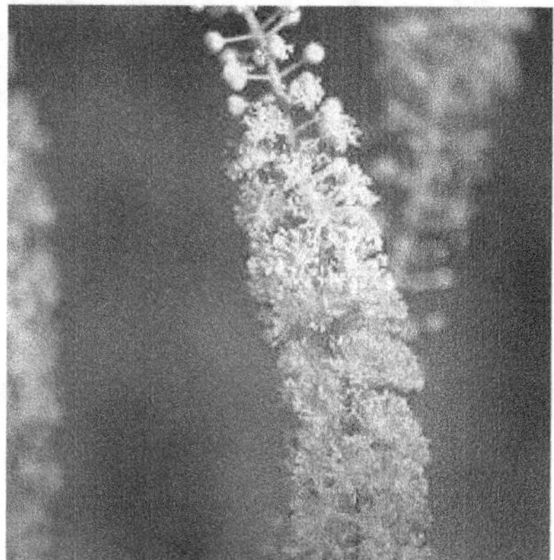

Black Cohosh

Black Cohosh is an herb and is plant based and it helps with muscle and nerve functions. It's wonderful for aches and pains and relieves menopause and andropause. Black Cohosh helps to prevent weight gain, hot flashes and night sweats. It prevents inflammation so if that is what you're suffering from have some Black Cohosh. It helps to relive a sore throat, you can take this if you're congested, and, if you have high blood pressure this will do wonders for you. Do you know that you can take for a snake bite? It's good for heart disease, brain disease, and crows feet. If you are having menstrual problems please take some Black Cohosh. Black Cohosh helps with arthritis, gout, depression, and anxiety. This helps to induce your labor if you are over your due date, but ask your doctor first. It also increases the chance of pregnancy. It regulates your blood sugar which is great if you are diabetic. Want undisturbed sleep, take some Black Cohosh. Black Cohosh improves healing after a bone fracture. It helps to prevent blood clots and guess what, HIV.

Chapter 4
 Vegetables

Eating vegetables boosts the immune system and have many benefits. They are full of vitamins and minerals which we all need, so eat all of your vegetables. Try to eat a variety of them because there are so many of them out there. There are Indian and Asian vegetables that are healthy to eat as well you should always try something new.

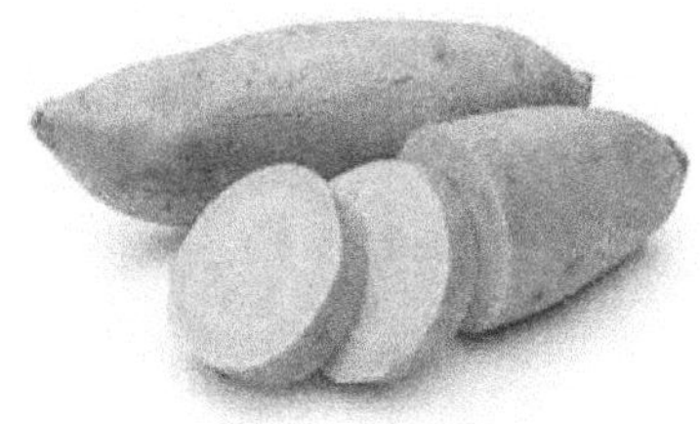

Sweet potato is good for your heart, brain, bones, your nervous system and lungs. It has the whole vitamin B complex and is much healthier than white potato.

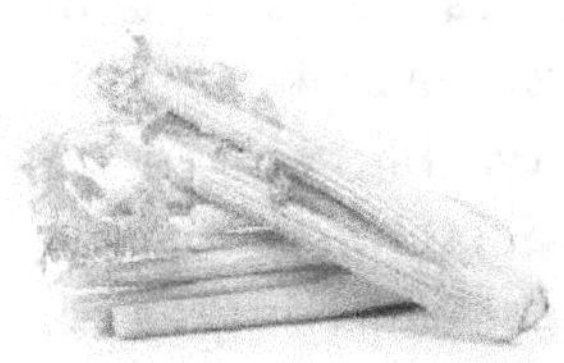

Celery lowers your blood pressure, helps with weight loss, and reduces inflammation. Celery helps to reduce stress and aids in restful sleep so if you're suffering with insomnia, you should try eating celery. It helps to prevent cancer and it boosts your sexual drive. Okay men, start eating some celery. It's good for your eye health and it reduces menstrual discomfort. Eating celery reduces bad cholesterol and aids with your digestion.

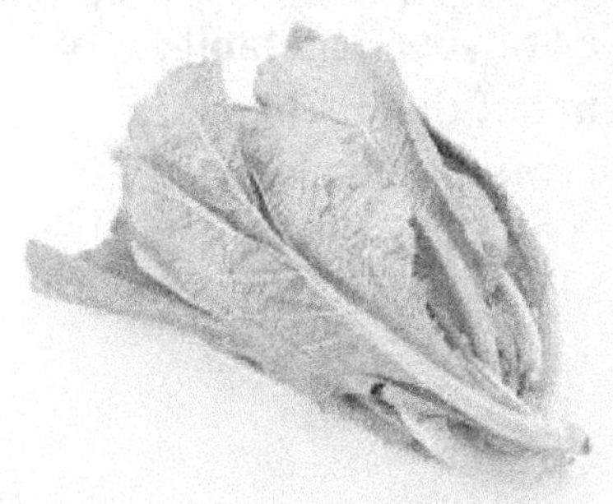

Mustard Greens helps with the flu and viruses. It detoxifies the liver and helps with bone mass. It's good for arthritis, your vision, your skin, and your eyes. Having mood swings eat some mustard greens. It is great if you want help with your memory and your thoughts. Women, eat these green to helps to regulate your

menstrual cycle. It's great for pregnant women, and helps to fight cancer. It also contains vitamin B.

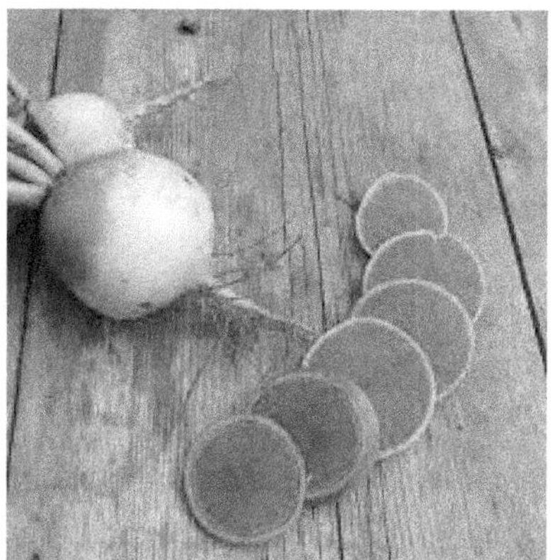

Radish

Radish helps if you have a cold, cough, the flu, or any virus. It helps with your kidneys, your thyroids, and your heart. Eating radishes help your bones, gall bladder, and your liver. Radishes are good for your hair and your skin. Eat radishes if you're running a fever. They are great for your brain and helps with mood swings. They are great in improving your thinking and helps with your digestive system. It has vitamins A, E, K, iron, zinc, magnesium, calcium, and folic acid.

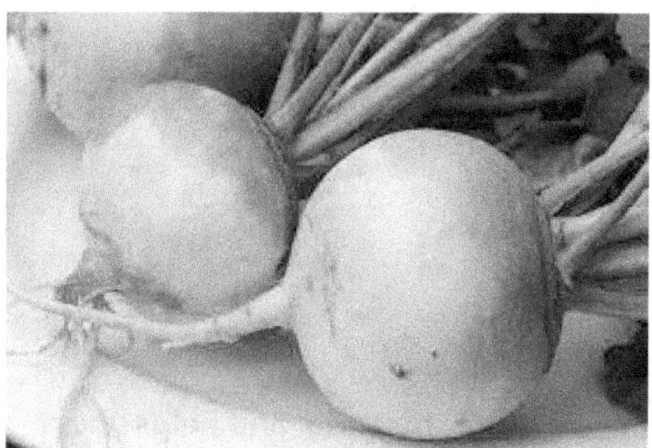

Turnips

Turnips are good to eat if you have a cold, a cough, a virus or the flu. It's great vegetable to eat if you suffer with asthma. It helps your respiratory system, your heart, and your eyes. It helps to prevent inflammation and swelling in your body. Eating turnips helps your blood, and your digestion. These greens are great for your bones and arthritis. They help to fight cancer, and helps to prevent tumors. It helps with weight loss and gives you energy. It has vitamins C, B9, and K.

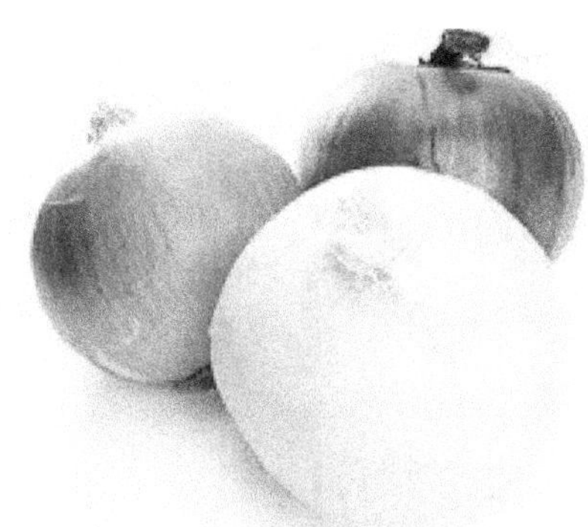

<u>Onions</u>

Onions helps to regulate your blood sugar and blood pressure. If you're diabetic include onions in your diet. Onions helps with diarrhea and it helps to fight cancer. If you or anyone you know has cancer, tell them to incorporate onions into their meals Onions. Contain vitamin C which helps to fight colds, the flu and coughs. It reduces inflammation, heals infections, and increases sperm count. Let's jump on these onions fellows. It prevents tooth decay an reduces tooth pain. You can actually place onions on your aching tooth to ease the pain. Onions eliminates worms in your stomach. It reduces pain and inflammation the joints, and is an antiseptic and an antibiotic, they also help if you have an ear-ache.

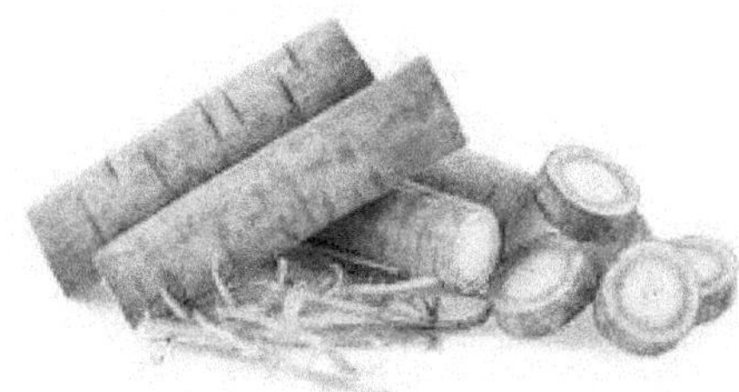

<u>Burdock</u>

Burdock detoxifies your body. It helps to eliminates gut bacteria, and helps your kidneys. Burdock is beneficial for your stomach. It helps to relieve cramps, gout, arthritis, and chest pain. It's great for your heart, regulates your blood sugar which makes it great for diabetics and is good for burns and hormonal imbalance. Burdock also fights cancer.

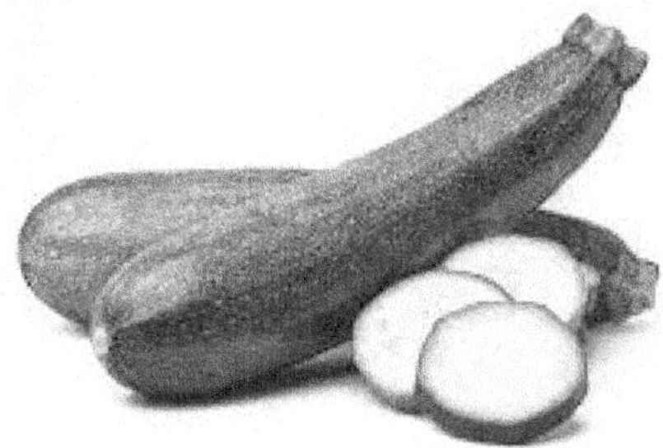

Zucchini has vitamins A, K, the B complex, C magnesium, collagen, potassium and calcium. It's low in calories, low in starch, high in fiber, and it hydrates your body. Zucchini regulates your blood pressure, is good for coughs, colds, the flu and viruses. It helps to slow down the aging process, now who doesn't want that to slow down. Are you looking to lose some weight, eat zucchini. If you're going through depression eating some zucchini can really help with that . Zucchini is good for infections and they help to hydrate your hair. Its good for your bones and your thyroids. Eating Zucchini is one way to prevent mood swings so it's a great addition to your diet if you are going through menopause. They help to regulate your blood sugar making it great for diabetics. If you or someone you know is experiencing heart problems, zucchini is the way to go. It helps to fight cancer and is great to eat if you have colon or prostate cancer. Zucchini is good for your mental health, your bones, teeth and your skin. This is a great vegetable to eat if you are pregnant .

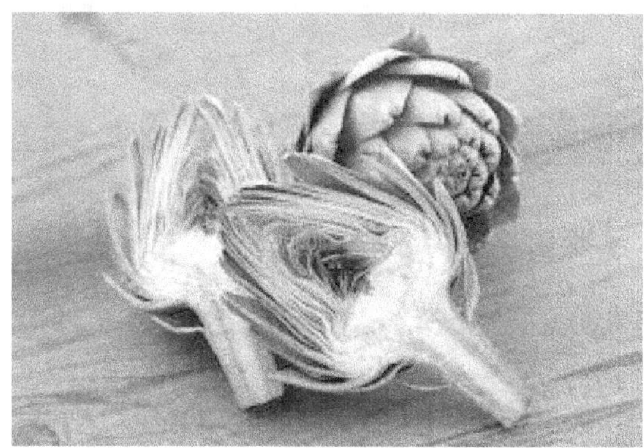

Artichokes have vitamins B, K, E, magnesium, zinc, potassium, calcium and iron. They give you a healthy liver and helps with your digestion. It's good for bone health, gout, joint pain, and arthritis. They're great to eat for your heart health and helps to fight cancer. Artichoke treat diabetes and help with Alzheimer and Dementia. They regulate your cholesterol and lowers your blood pressure. It's good for cough, colds, the flu and viruses.

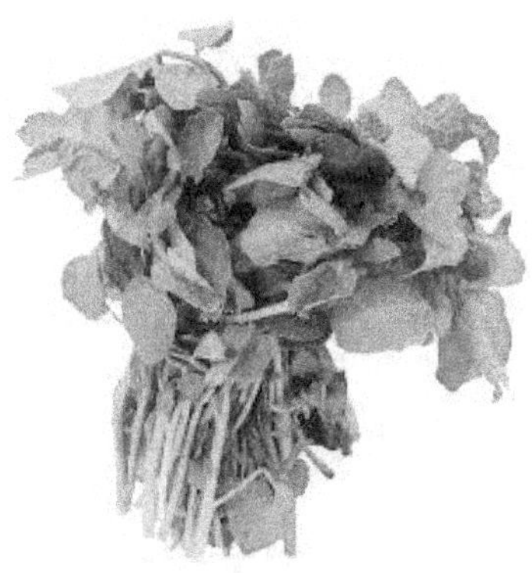

<u>Watercress</u>

Watercress contains vitamins B1, C, E, B6, zinc, iron, magnesium, B12, A and iodine. Watercress is good for your brain, liver, skin, hair, nails, and your kidneys. It's good for the health of your heart and bones. It strengthens your red blood cells helps to fight memory loss so if you or someone you know has Alzheimer or Dementia add watercress to their diet. Watercress fights bacteria, and it helps to fight depression. They are good for your eyes and are great if you are suffering with night vision. They help to fight infections and viruses making it great for the corona virus. It breaks up kidney and bladder stones and helps to remove phlegm.

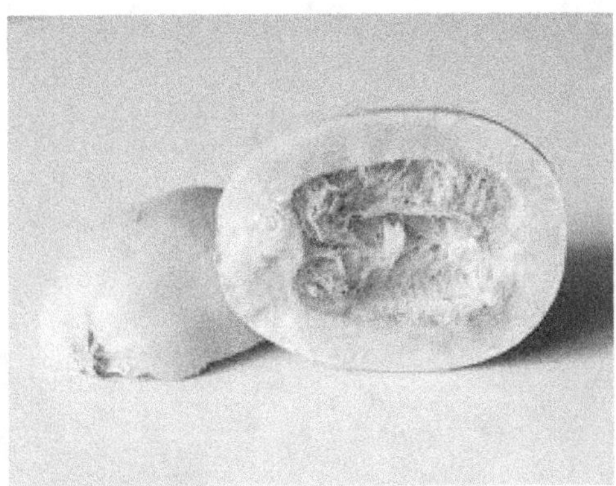

<u>Spaghetti Squash</u>

Spaghetti squash has vitamins A, C, E, the B complex, iron, magnesium zinc, potassium, omega3 and fiber. It's good for your eyes and helps to regulate your bowels. Spaghetti squash is good for your stomach, your skin, hair, and nails. They are great to eat for the improvement of your joints. It assists with weight loss, is good for gut health and brain health so it's a great vegetable to eat for those suffering with Alzheimer's. It's good for bone health, strokes, colds, the flu and coughs. It helps to prevent heart attacks and memory loss. It combats inflammation and may help with the reduction of birth defects. Spaghetti squash lowers the blood pressure and helps to prevent breast cancer. It balances out your hormones, stabilizes your moods and helps to fight depression. If you become weary and your brain don't seem to be operating well, eat some spaghetti squash.

It aids in your digestion, it treats arthritis and its good for people suffering with Alzheimer. It opens up and cleans your arteries. It treats skin disorders, and strengthens your muscles and tissues. It lowers your cholesterol and decreases stress and anxiety and also helps to fight multiple scoliosis.

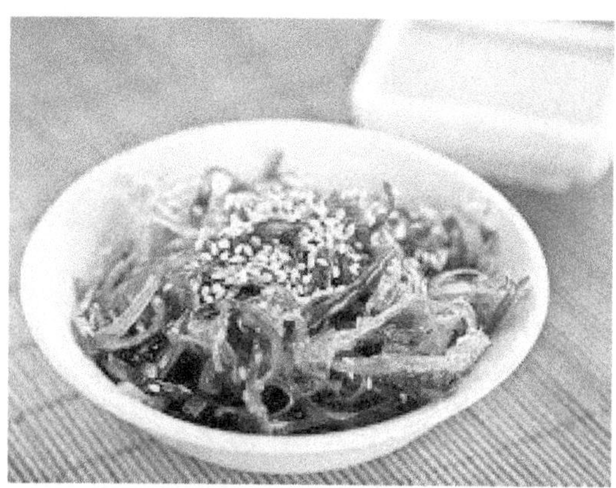
Kelp

Kelp has vitamins A, C, D, iron, zinc, calcium, B and K. Kelp regulates your metabolism, it has iodine and is a seaweed. It is good for your thyroids and has fat fighting properties which helps with weight loss. Did you know that eating kelp prevents diabetes, helps with blood disorders and blood clots? Kelp prevents strokes and heart attacks. It's great for your brain and helps to boost your energy. Kelp is good for the brain making it great for Alzheimer and Dementia. It helps if you're anemic, it builds up your bones, it protects from radiation and removes radiation from the body. It helps to fight cancer, heals the liver and is good for your cell membrane. It's good to help prevent stress, inflammation and tumors. It also makes you happier.

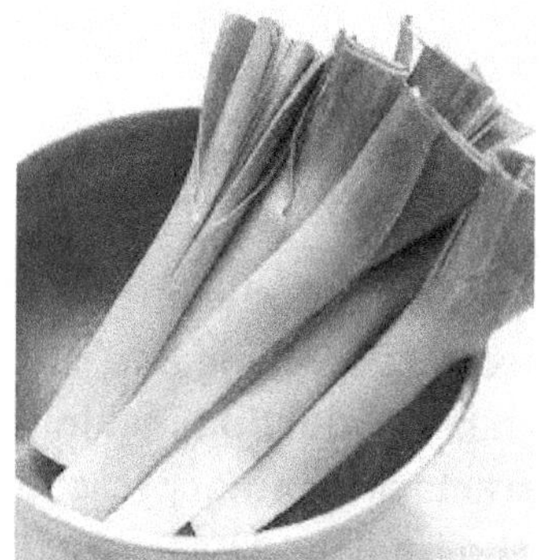
Leeks

Leeks contains vitamins C, B6, A, calcium and minerals. It lowers and controls your blood pressure. Leeks fights cancer, eliminates uric acid from your body and gives you a healthy nervous system. It's good for you if you're anemic and It's good for your digestion and your brain. It helps to prevent memory loss and it increases your concentration. Leeks reduces intestinal bloating and helps to prevent brain defects Eating leeks will be very beneficial for pregnant women. It helps to protect your heart and cleanses the colon, this is a natural laxative. It helps with inflammation, swelling and urination and helps to regulate your cholesterol level.

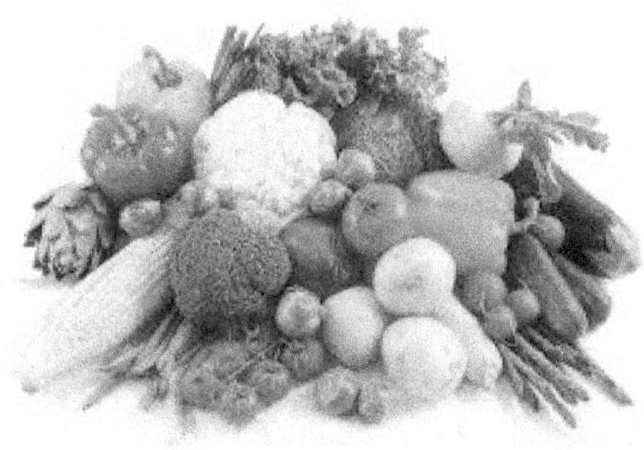

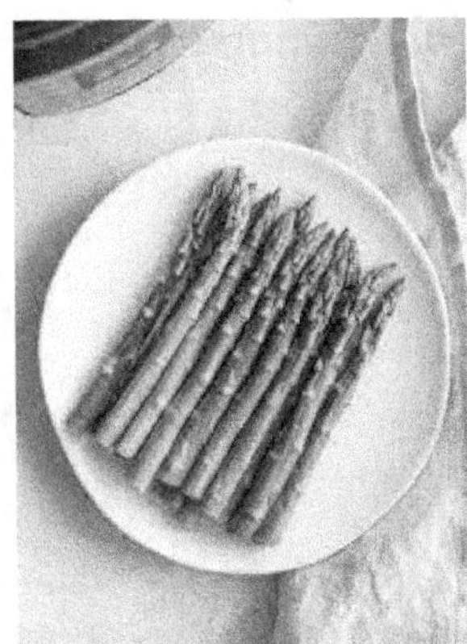

Asparagus

Asparagus lowers the blood pressure, dissolves kidney stones, it fights chronic fatigue syndrome, helps to prevent arthritis and gout and reduces swelling and inflammation. It has vitamins A, C, K and B12. It stimulates hair production making it thicker and much more manageable. It helps to fight cataracts and urinary tract infection. Asparagus helps to cure colon cancer, it alkaline the body and has protein. It helps to prevent diabetes, helps with your sex drive and is an aphrodisiac. Its an anti-fungal and anti-viral. It's good for colds, viruses, the flu and coughs. This vegetable is a natural laxative. It reduces diseases and is good to eat if you have varicose veins. It alkaline the blood and detoxes the entire body. It helps the brain and helps to manage Alzhiemer's Disease and Dementia. It helps to improve your memory. Asparagus helps to fight lung and breast cancer, its a brain booster, it gives you energy and helps to prevent birth defects.

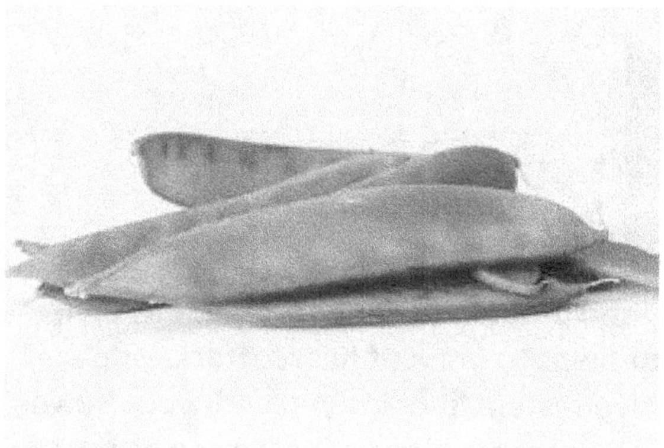

Snow peas has vitamins C, iron, fiber, omega3, folate acid and magnesium. They help your bones and improves your brain health and build great brain cells. Snow peas helps with the development of the fetus. They help to prevent asthma, cures diarrhea and it lowers heart attacks and strokes. They help to eliminate sleep disorders and is good for your skin, eyes and your gut health.

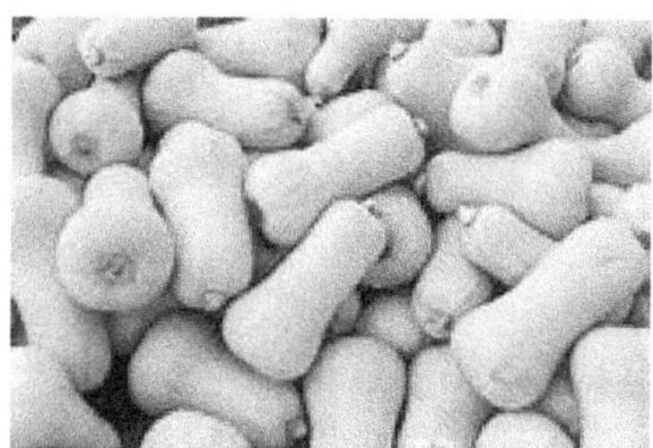

Butternut Squash helps to fight heart disease and obesity. It has vitamins C, A, B6, E, iron, zinc, folate, collagen and calcium. It helps to regulate your blood sugar making it great for diabetics. It's good for type 1 diabetes. It lowers and prevents high blood pressure and is good for your skin, hair, and nails. Butter squash strengthens your bones and prevents swelling and fatigue. It helps with brain health which makes it good for Alzheimer and Dementia. If you know someone with these diseases, tell them to start to incorporate butternut squash into their diet. It gives you energy and helps to prevent anemia. It's great for your digestive system.

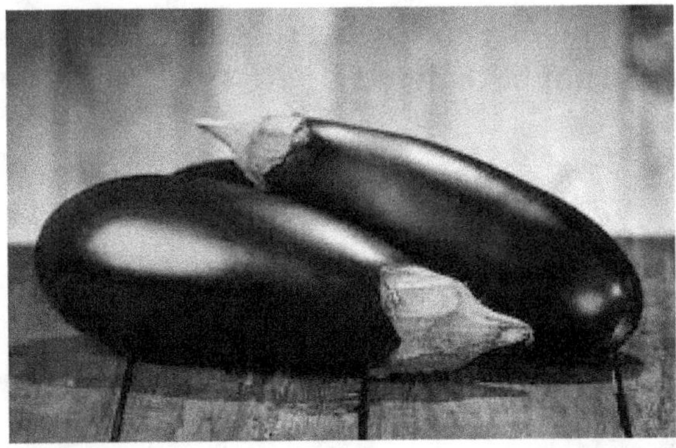

Eggplant has calcium, magnesium, folate, and potassium. It has vitamins A, C, K, and the whole B complex. Eating egg plant helps to prevent heart attacks and strokes. It helps to promote a good digestive system. It helps you with your bowel movement, nourishes your brain cells and it prevents blood clots. Eating eggplant regulates your blood pressure, improves your skin and manages the cholesterol levels in your body. It keeps your bones from deteriorating and it's good for your hair. It prevents birth defects and ladies, it helps to regulate your menstrual cycle.

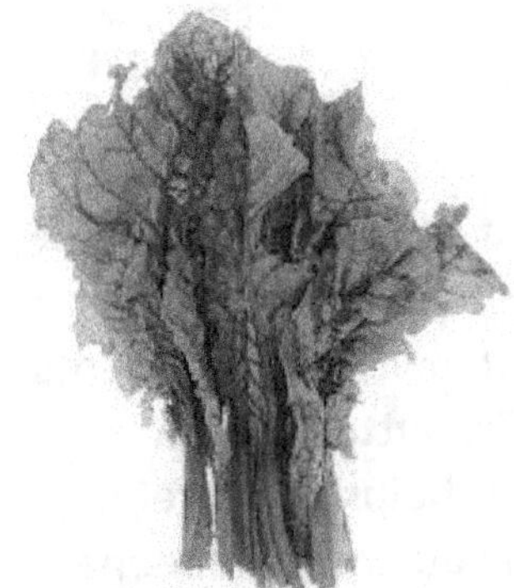

Swiss Chard has vitamins K, C, E, iron, zinc, calcium, magnesium, B1, and B3, and protein. It helps to prevent cancer and stabilizes your blood sugar which helps to treat diabetes so its great for diabetics. It boosts your brain power and helps to prevent memory loss. It helps to fight colon cancer and Alzheimer. Swiss chard helps to fight liver damage, and reduces muscle cramps. It stimulates bone growth and bone development.

Chapter 5

The Effects Of Your Emotions

Did you know that your emotions can boost the immune system and have many benefits? Your emotions can affect your day and the people around you in a profound way. Our emotions can either strengthen us or drain us of our senses. Your emotions can elevate you or have you sitting in the corner banging your head against a wall. Watching a movie, hearing a song even things that you see can all affect you emotionally.

Joy

Being joyful actually boosts your immune system. Who would have known that being joyful can do that? Joy lengthens your life span and can help to you sleep better. It drives out discouragement and has the tendency to draw people to you. Joy also strengthens relationships.

Laughter

Laughter boosts the immune system. It releases hormones to make you feel better. It's good for your lungs, muscles, and your mood. It helps to fight anxiety and depression. Laughter is great for your mental health and your blood. It helps to fight cancer and it brings you peace of mind. Laughter can help to keep you calm and gives you so much comfort. It also helps with fighting ailments. It can help to lower your fear factor and it lowers the acid in your body. Laughter helps you to focus and gives you a sense of awareness and alertness. It detoxes your organs, and supplies fresh blood.

Anger

Anger weakens your liver. It makes you depressed and irritable. Anger makes you hard to get along with and will cause you to become bitter. You can begin to hate yourself and those around you.

Worry

Worrying weakens your stomach causing ulcers, and ulcers are contagious.

Fear

Fear will give you pains in your stomach and will weaken your kidneys. Fear also gives you pains in your sides.

Chapter 6

Foods To Avoid And Foods That Heals

Sugary drinks, powdered lemonade, aspartame (this is a sugar substitute, always check the ingredients to make sure this is not included), coca-cola and sugary cereal are foods to stay away from. When you finish a box of cereal, look at all of the sugar that's left. Did you know that coca-cola can remove acid build up on car batteries? If it can do that, imagine what it can do to your body. These things has no health benefits what so ever.

Foods That Lowers The Blood Pressure
This is a list of foods that lowers the blood pressure, garlic, berries, apples, celery, yogurt, kale, avocado, banana, mustard greens, turnip greens, lemon, spinach (spinach is not good for bone pain, gout or if you have arthritis), sweet potato, grapes, onion, mint leaves, watermelon, cayenne pepper, salmon, sardines, nuts, seeds, olive oil, brown rice, black rice, barley, papaya and water.

Foods That Heals
You can eat these foods foods for healing your body;
Kidneys, cranberries, red peppers, blueberries, strawberries, onions, garlic, cabbage, cauliflower, red grapes, salmon, celery, burdock, parsley.
Avoid - Sugary and salty foods, cold cuts, processed meats, tomato, cocoa powder, tofu, potato, yam, dried fruit, avocado, banana, milk, yogurt, oranges, orange juice, beans and honey dew melon.

Diabetics should eat these foods to help to regulate their blood sugar-
Kale, barley grass, and avocado.
And these are foods for diabetics to avoid - Soda, bacon, white rice, flour, pancakes, dried foods, ketchup, hamburgers and bananas.

Here are foods to help if you have cancer or know anyone who does-
Blackberries, raspberries, onion, leafy greens vegetables, kale, Tumeric (this is a spice), artichoke, garlic, tomato, olive oil, dark chocolate, oregano oil (this oil builds up your immune system), cauliflower, brussel sprout, avocado, broccoli, mushroom, ginseng and watermelon.

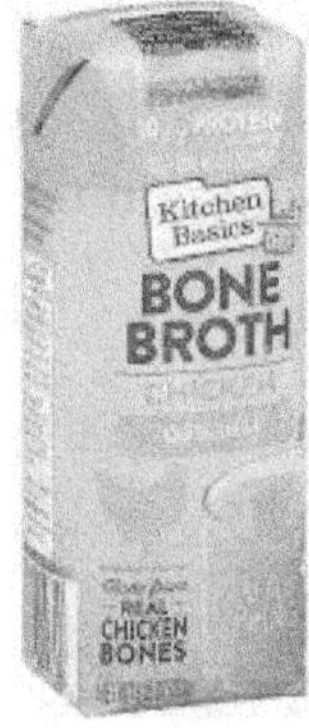

Bone Broth
Bone broth fights liver cancer, repairs bone growth and increases your red blood cells and your blood count. Bone broth absorbs calcium and other minerals. It detoxes the body and are healthy for your kidneys. It's great for diabetics. It helps to fight fatigue and diarrhea. Bone broth fights food sensitivity and assist in weight loss. It helps with vomiting and it keeps you body from becoming weak and it helps you to focus.

Here are some healing things that we never thought about can heal and are quite enjoyable to do.

Music

Music reduces stress and anxiety. It has the ability to drive out depression and will make you well in your spirit, soul and body. But the wrong music can make you sick because music goes into the inner part of your soul. The right music such as gospel music creates creative thinking , enhances your blood vessel functions and releases your serotonin. Music is good for your brain and lowers your blood pressure. It has the ability to relax you and can help you to eat less. Music is great therapy for those who has cancer because it has a healing effect, especially the harp. Music stimulates the brain and is great for stroke patients. It also improves your coordination. Music is wonderful for unborn babies. It boosts your memory and lifts your mood. Music improves reading and math skills and it improves your quality of sleep. It motivates you and decreases pain. Music increases the rate of healing, it helps you to run faster, walk longer, swim faster and bike longer. Believe it or not, music improves your immune system.

A Sing-A-Long

Amazingly a sing-a-long is good for your heart. It lowers your blood pressure, improves your lungs, and respiratory system. It can help with your breathing and is good for your mental health. Its good for your blood circulation and your overall health and well being. It builds up your confidence and self-esteem. It's wonderful to do when you exercise. It helps to give you a longer life span, increases your morality and induces happiness and joy. It improves the brain function, increases your IQ and enhances your intelligence and your mood. A sing-a-long releases serotonin, endorphins and increases your immune system. A sing-a-long leads to a happy life. Imagine sitting in a waiting room when all of a sudden people start singing. It increases social behavior and helps to bond people together. It gives you energy and relives anxiety and depression.

Reading

Reading lowers stress and anxiety. Reading slows your heart beat, eases muscle tension, gives you a sense of well being, enhances social skills, increases life span, boosts longevity, boosts intelligence and increases your IQ. Reading improves your sleep, stimulates your brain and helps to fight brain disease. Reading alters your state of mind, improves your concentration, helps with your memory and helps you to focus at lot more. It increases your vocabulary and broadens it as well. You learn to spell better and it helps you to pronounce words. Reading expands your knowledge and helps you to develop your imagination because you can actually travel to many places in your mind when you read. Reading helps with creating your activity and has the ability to increases your faith. It also helps you to obey. It strengthens you spiritually, gives you stamina, sharpens your conviction and strengthens your commitment.

Pumpkins makes you feel good,
Blueberries changes your mood,
Coconut gives you a feeling of balance,
Chia seeds lifts up your energy,
Avocado gives you energy,
Swiss chard gives you energy,
Spinach gives you energy,
Water gives you energy and helps with depression and anxiety,
Walnuts help with depression and anxiety.

Chapter 7

Juicing And Smoothies

Juicing boosts the immune system especially since it extracts all of the vitamins, minerals, and nutrients out of fruits and vegetables.

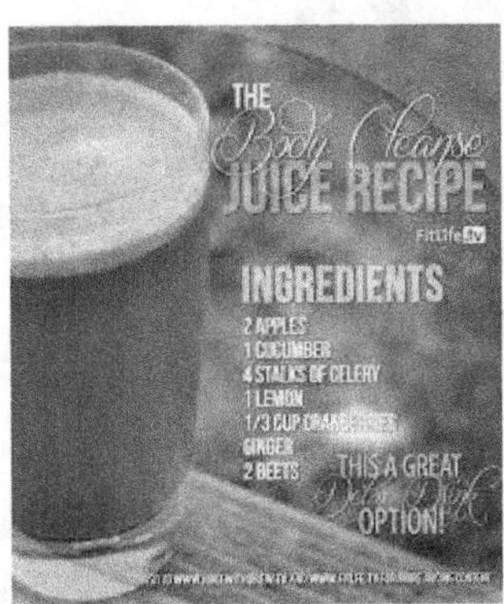

Celery Juicing

Celery has vitamin C. It flushes out your system and helps to prevent bloating and cancer. It reduces stress, depression and mood swings. Celery juicing helps to prevent constipation. It fights insomnia and is good if you have arthritis or gout. It helps to remove bone pain and helps to prevent memory loss. It's good for gut health, it calms your nerves, fights infections and detoxes the body. Celery juicing helps with your thyroids and the urinary tract. It renews your mind and brain cells.

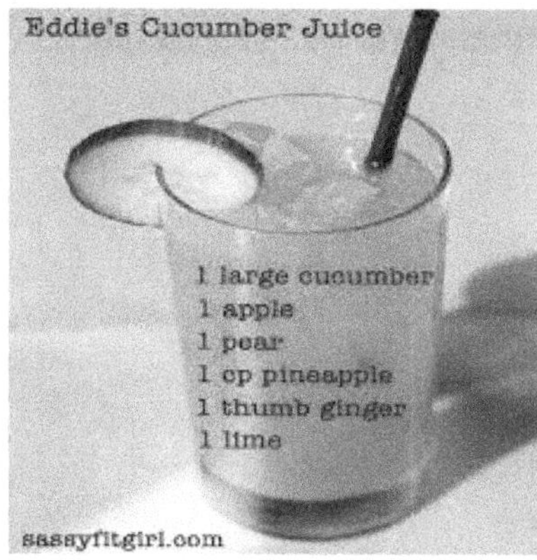

Cucumber Juicing

Cucumbers hydrates your body. It helps you to urinate, lowers your blood pressure, reduces hunger pains, reduces fat and detoxifies your whole system. It regulates your blood sugar and balances out your hormones.

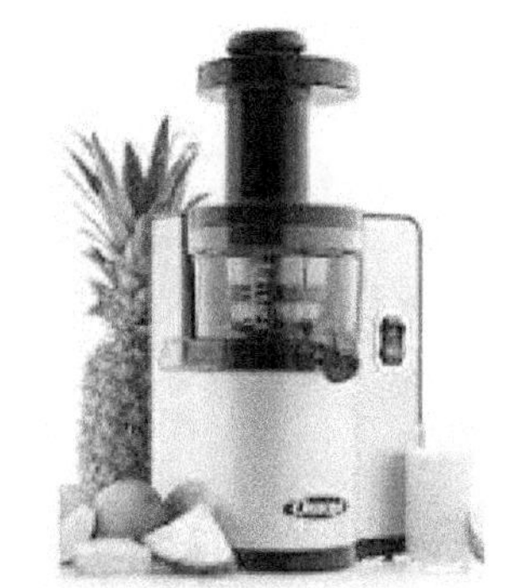

Omega

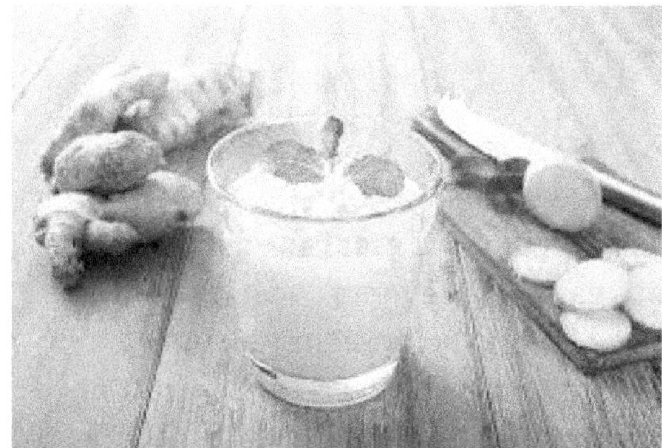

Ginger Juicing

Ginger juice regulates your blood pressure. It helps with your digestive system, reduces pain and is good for your hair. It fights colds, the flu and viruses. Ginger juice is great for your kidneys, it prevents heart burn and helps to prevent prostate cancer. This is great to drink for women going through morning sickness. It

cleanses your urinary tract and it helps to fight colon cancer and ovarian cancer. It also reduces phlegm.

1/2 lb fresh ginger root (about one cup full)
1/4 cup lemon juice
Pinch salt (Himalayan Salt)
3/4 cup Stevia
5 cups water divided

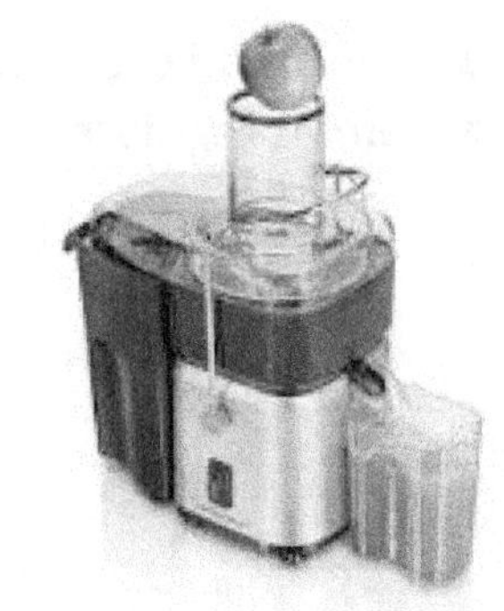
Hamilton Beach

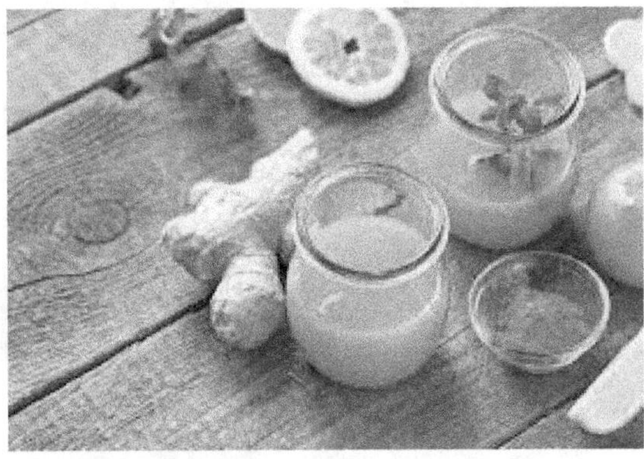

Tumeric Juicing

Tumeric juice helps to regulate your blood sugar making it great for diabetics. It's good for your brain health, helps to eliminate gas and prevents constipation. Tumeric juicing prevent blood clots and is good to help to prevent gout and arthritis. It helps to prevent strokes, increases your memory and concentration, and it supports good breast health. This juice it has vitamin C.

Ingredients

1 small orange	2 Tbs. Lemon juice
1 Tbs ginger	1 1/2 cups of water
1-2 inch Tumeric	

Now we come to the smoothies. Smoothies boosts the immune system and have many benefits. You can put just about anything in a smoothie.

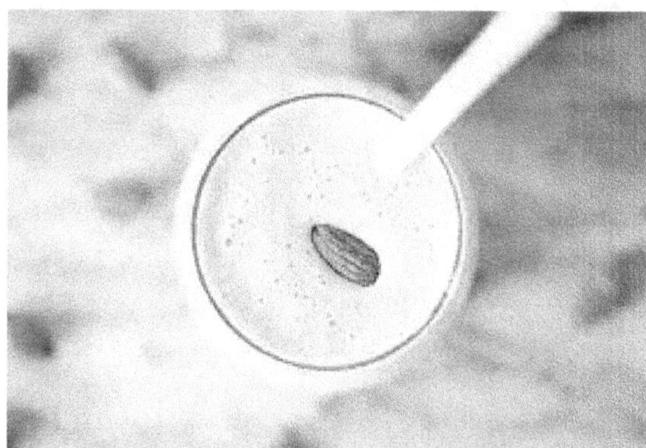

Almond Milk Smoothie

Almond mild smoothies helps with weight loss. It prevents cancer, helps to flush out the kidneys and is good for your bones, eyes, skin, and hair. This smoothie has Omega fatty acid along with vitamins A, B, and D.

1/2 cup almond milk
1/2 tsp vanilla extract
Banana peeled
1 Tbs peanut butter or almond butter
1 cup ice cubes

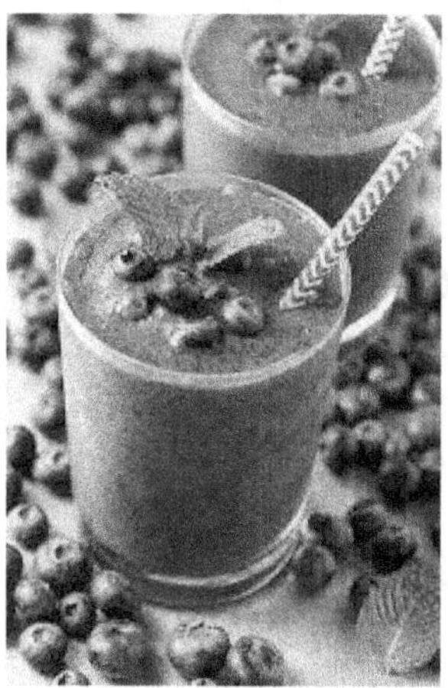

Blueberry Smoothie

Blueberry smoothies are good for mental health, Dementia, the brain, your memory, heart health and it aids in weight loss. Blueberry smoothies lowers your blood pressure and regulates your blood sugar making it a good smoothie for diabetics. It helps if your constipated. This smoothie fights colds, the flu, and viruses. It has vitamins C, the B complex and iron. it helps your nerves, and it fights cancer cells.

1/4 cups blueberries fresh or frozen
1 medium ripe banana
1/2 medium orange peeled and quartered
3/4 to 1 cup Almond milk

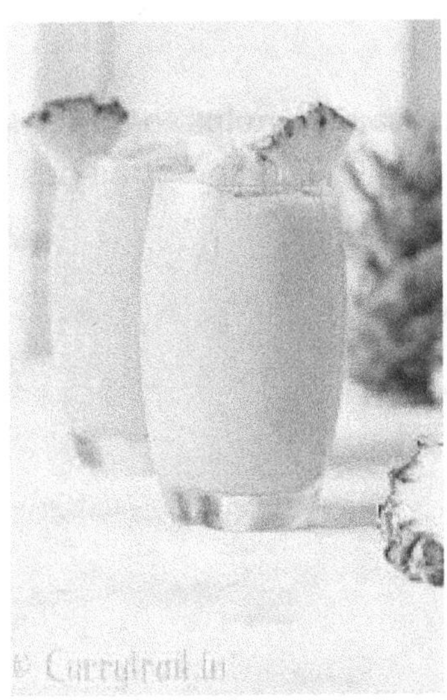

Pineapple Smoothie

Pineapple smoothies are a natural detox. It boosts your energy level, is good for your brain, kidneys, thyroids, teeth, vision and your sinuses. It helps to fight arthritis and gout and is wonderful to drink to support your bones. Drinking this smoothie is good for your skin. It helps to get rid of worms and parasites. It assists in weight loss and helps if you are suffering with constipation because it helps to regulate your bowels. It helps to fight cancer, is good for your mental health and your heart health. It regulates your blood pressure, it great to drink if you or someone you know is suffering with Dementia because it improves memory loss. It helps you to concentrate more and helps helps to fight bacterial infections. This smoothie has vitamins C, and B.

Ingredients
1 cup ice cubes
2 cups frozen pineapple chunks or fresh pineapple
1/2 cup banana
1/2 cup plain Greek yogurt
3/4 cup pineapple juice

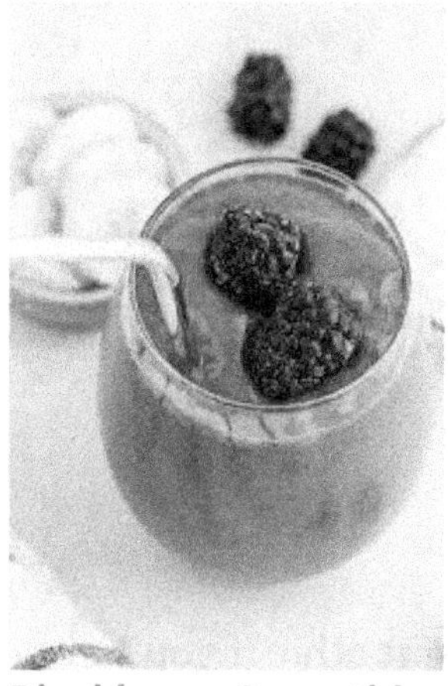

Blackberry smoothies helps with weight loss, prevents cancer, cleanse the blood, is good for bone health, gout and arthritis. It is low in sugar making it great for diabetics, it's good for your skin and your colon. This smoothie is great for the brain, it helps with your bowels, mood swings and depression. It fights colds, the flu and coughs. It also has vitamins B9, B5,B3, B2, magnesium, and iron.

Ingredient

3/4 cup frozen or fresh blackberries
1/2 cup frozen pineapple chunks
1/2 cup plain Greek yogurt
1 cup almond milk
1 Tbs honey

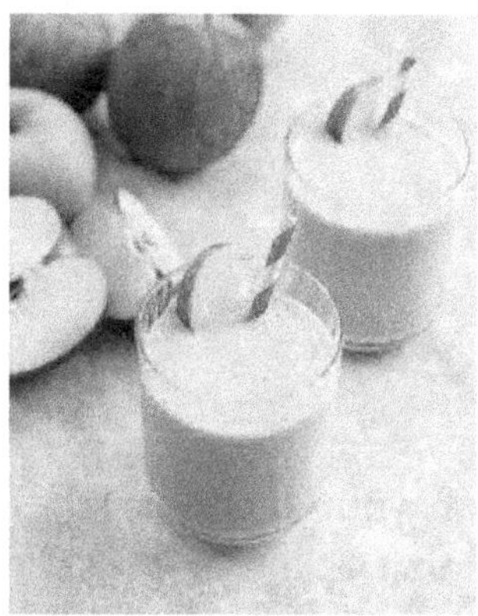

Apple smoothies are good for your teeth, gums, bones, arthritis, gout, constipation, mood swings and weight loss. It reduces strokes, is good for your heart, brain, and has vitamins A, B6, and C.

Ingredient

1 large apple peeled, cored and chopped
1/2 cup almond milk
1/3 cup plain Greek yogurt
5 almonds
1 tsp honey

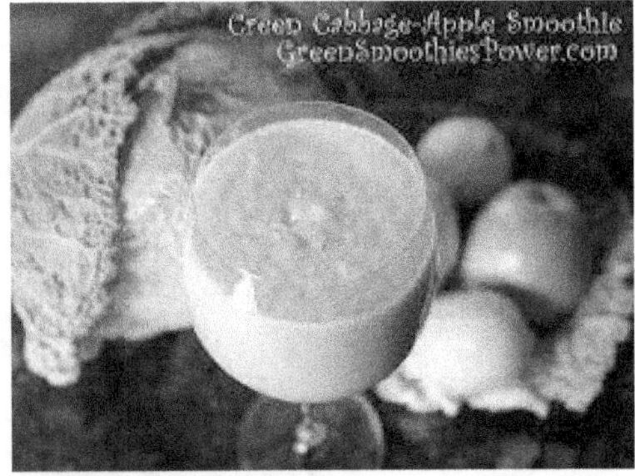

Cabbage Smoothie

Cabbage smoothies helps to fight yeast infections. Drink this smoothie if you have asthma it is good for that. Cabbage smoothie has vitamins and minerals and it helps to fight stomach cancer. It's a great smoothie to drink for weight loss. It detoxes the liver, fights lung cancer, colon cancer,and stomach cancer.

Ingredient

2 cups green cabbage
1 banana
1 apple

1 Tbs almonds
1/2 cups oats
2 1/2 cups almond milk, coconut milk or filtered water
1 lemon wedge

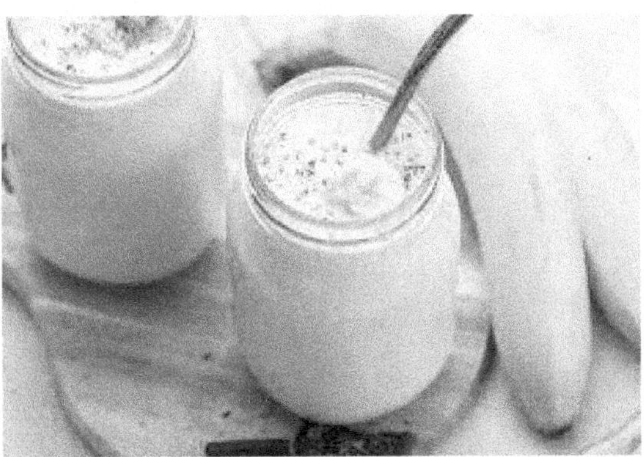

Banana Smoothie

Banana smoothies helps to lower the blood pressure. It boosts your energy level, stops muscle cramps, regulates your bowels, is good for morning sickness, depression, your kidneys, mood swings, and helps with diarrhea. This smoothie is not intended for diabetics.

Ingredients

1/4 cup honey
3/4 tsp pure vanilla extract
2 medium ripe banana
1 1/2 cups Greek yogurt
1/2 cup ice

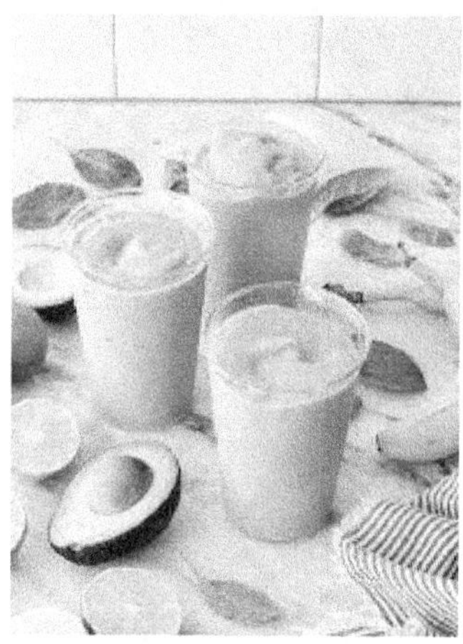

Avocado smoothies helps to fight cancer. It has vitamins B17, K, E, C, B6, iron, zinc, folate, and potassium. An avocado smoothie lowers cholesterol, absorbs nutrients and is good for your heart and skin. This smoothie lowers your blood pressure, is a good mouthwash, and is good for the liver. It lowers blood sugar making it good for Diabetics, it's good for your digestion, and it helps to fight food cravings.

Ingredients
1 cup Almond milk
1/2 Avocado
1 Banana
1-2 Tbs Honey
Blend and enjoy

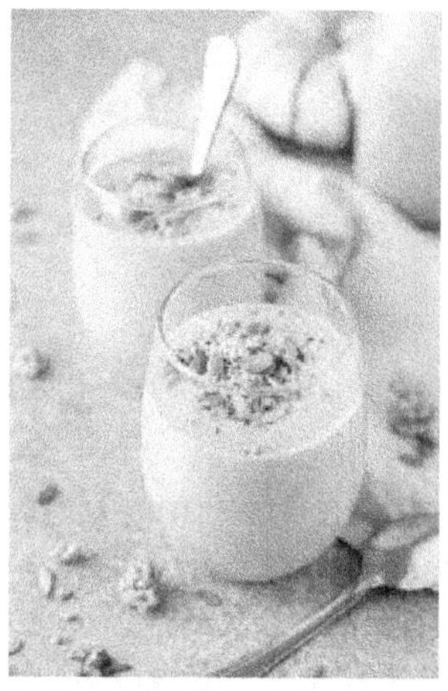

Pumpkin smoothies promotes heart health, liver health, kills parasites, regulates blood sugar making it good for diabetics, it has vitamins K, E, zinc, magnesium, Omega 3, it's and anti-viral preventive, pumpkin seeds helps to prevent kidney stones, depression, insomnia giving you peaceful sleep helping with your sleep cycle, it fights fungus, Prostate, lung, breast, and stomach cancers, it reduces the effect of type 2 Diabetes, it does wonders for your hair and nails plus it alkalizes the body.

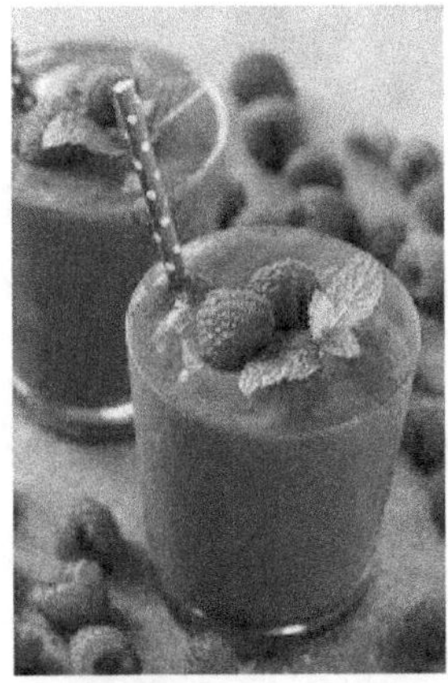

Raspberry smoothie prevents cancer, depression, mood swings, colds, coughs, the flu and viruses, it reduces stress and tension bringing you peace and calm in your mind, it helps gut health and your bowels, it also helps to keep your arteries open.

Ingredients

2 cups frozen raspberries
1 banana
1/4 cup Greek yogurt
1/2 cup purified water
1/2 cup almond milk
1 Tbs honey

1/2 cup ice
Frozen raspberry and mint leaf for garnish

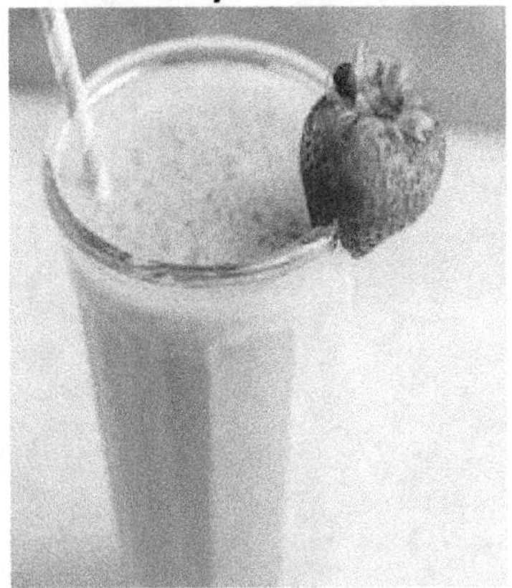

Strawberry smoothies helps to fight Prostate Cancer, it has vitamin C making it great for fighting colds, and the flu, it prevents strokes, allergies, and depression. It's good for your bones, helping to fight arthritis and gout. Strawberry Smoothies are good for your heart, your hair, wrinkles, constipation, and it burns fat, it also regulates your blood pressure.

Ingredients

2 lbs fresh strawberries
1 cup plain Greek yogurt
1/4 cup Almond milk

1/3 cup fresh pineapple
1/2 cup ice

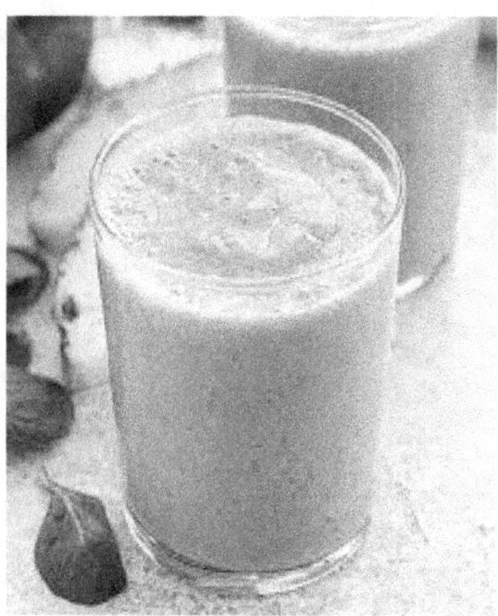

Spinach smoothies lowers the risk of cancer, it regulates your blood pressure, is good for your bones, skin, hair and nails, it gives you're a healthy brain, alkaline the body, help prevent heart disease, heart attacks, strokes, and constipation, it's good for your digestion and your blood, it's and anti-aging, it has vitamins B6, A, k, magnesium, iron and Omega3. It's full of fiber and gives you energy.

Ingredients

1 cup ice
2 cups frozen or fresh pineapple chunks
1/2 cup banana frozen or fresh
1 cup diced apples
2 cups baby spinach
1/2 cup Greek yogurt
1 cup Almond milk

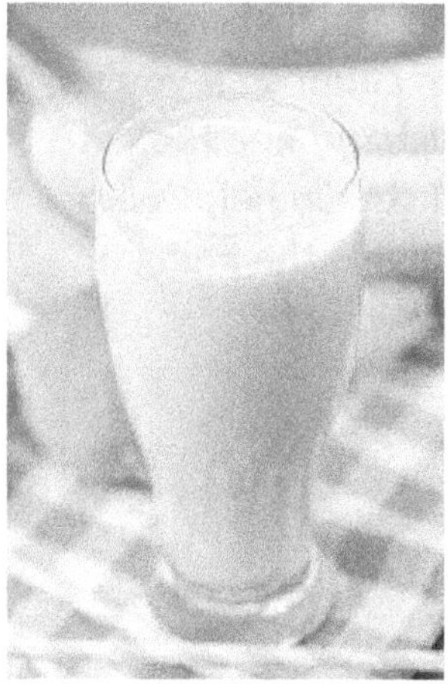

Peach smoothies has vitamins C and A, it has potassium and iron it kills parasites meaning it kills worms. It good for your nails, hair, skin, your urinary tract and your kidneys. It helps to regulate your blood pressure and cholesterol, it helps to prevent bone disorder, inflammation and swelling making it great to fight arthritis and gout, it's good for the nervous system and your bowels. It helps with weight loss, strokes, your kidneys and is good if you are anemic and is good for diabetics.

Ingredients

1 Banana
1 Peach
6 oz low fat peach yogurt
1/4 cup orange juice
1 cup ice

Chapter 8

Nuts

Nuts boost the immune system and have many benefits. Here is a list of a few of them.

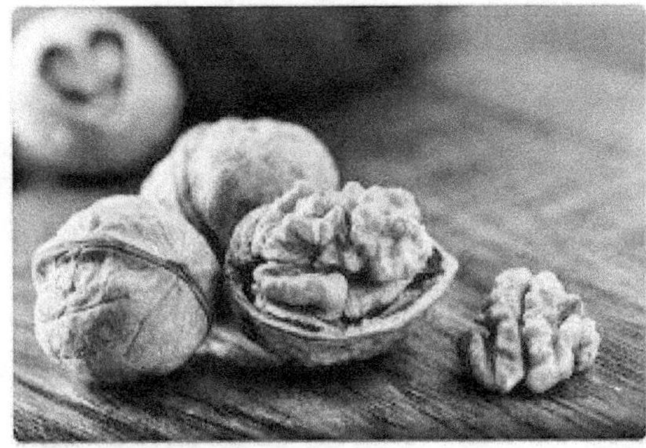

Walnuts

Walnuts helps to prevent inflammation, depression and cancer. They're good to eat if you are constipated. They are good to alleviate gout pain and arthritis. Walnuts reduces anxiety and stress. It helps to increase sperm count so if you're having a hard time getting pregnant women, you and your husband need to eat some walnuts. Its considered a super food for the brain, and actually helps with weight loss. It increases serotonin, and has protein. It also rebuilds the lining of your stomach.

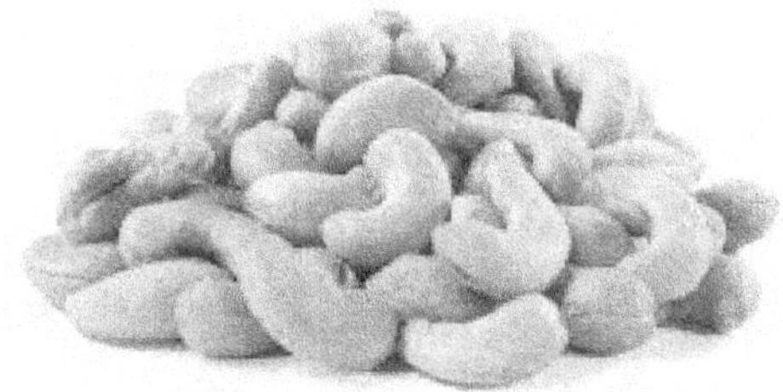

Cashews are good for your heart, they regulate your blood pressure and is good for your bones. Cashews helps to regulate your blood sugar making it great addition for a diabetics diet. It's good for your skin and hair and helps with the formation of your red blood cells. Cashews is a low carbohydrate diet. They have zinc, iron, copper, magnesium and vitamin B3.

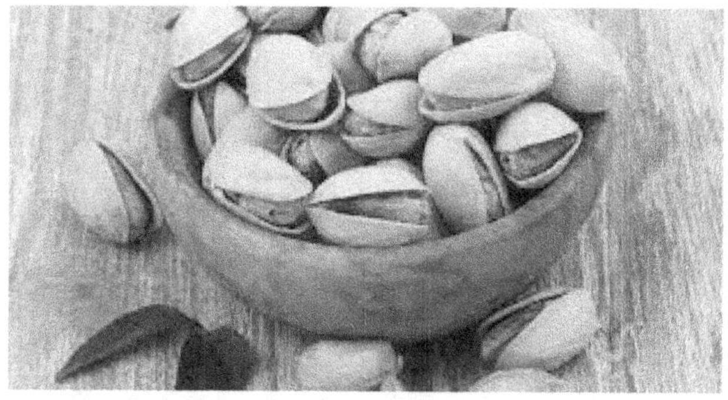

Pistachios helps to fight cancer and helps if you're constipated. Its an antidepressant and it's good for your well being. It helps with your emotions, it manages diabetes and it's good for building up your bone tissues. Pistachios helps with your blood pressure and digestion. It's good for coughs, colds, the flu and viruses. It's also good for a sore throat.

Chapter 9
Other Things That Boosts Your Immune System

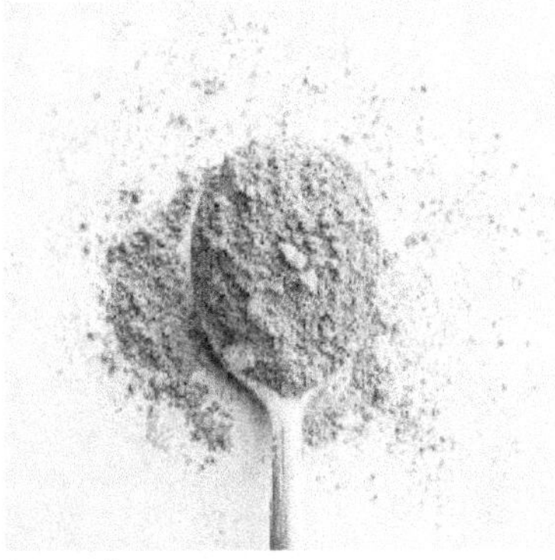

Matcha eliminates the chemicals in your body. It improves your memory and helps to fight Alzheimer and Dementia. It helps to fight brain diseases and improves your mood. It has Vitamins A, B, D, C, K and amino acid. Matcha is good for your skin, nails and hair. Matcha detoxes your body, lowers your cholesterol, reduces the risk of cancer and stress. It helps you to concentrate more, it boosts your metabolism and is good for colds, the flu, cough and viruses. It helps your heart, it burns fat, it helps with aging and is an anti fungal. It also has chlorophyll.

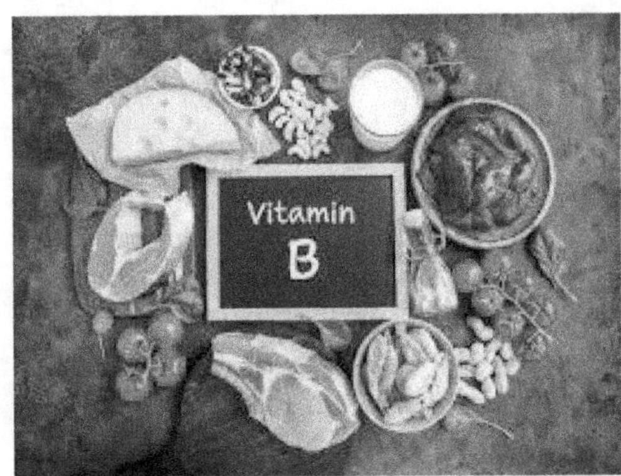

B Complex

The B complex of cause has vitamins B6 and B12, B3, and B9. It protects against heart and kidney disease. It prevent kidney stones and it helps to give proper function for your nervous system and your liver. The B complex can help with premenstrual pains and helps to maintain the function of your mind. It maintains a healthy level of hormones and helps to keep your blood vessels healthy. The B complex helps to treat skin diseases, acne, hair, dandruff and sickle cell anemia. It boosts your immune system and boosts your brain health. It regulates your sleep cycle, balances your blood sugar and helps hemoglobin to be carried throughout your blood system. It also helps the serotonin and dopamine in your body.

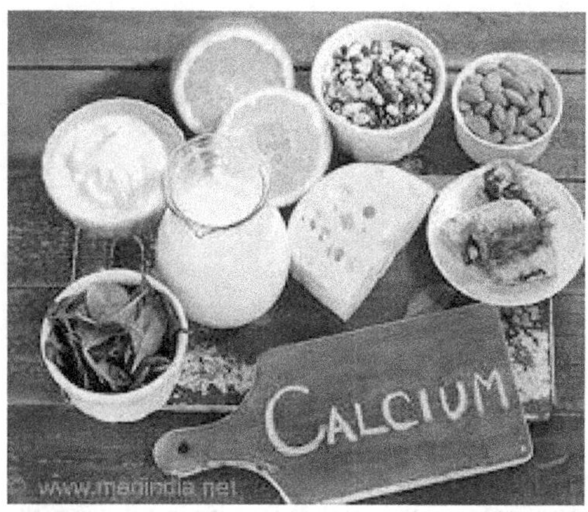

Calcium

Calcium helps to control your blood pressure. It reduces the chances of getting colon cancer and kidney stones. It's good for your bones and it helps to strengthen your heart. It helps to keep your blood from clotting and it alkaline your body. It's good for your nerves and your muscle functions. Calcium strengthens your teeth and gums and your bones. Calcium aids in the transportation of the nutrients in your body, it reduces PMS, decreases diabetes and boosts fertility.

Calcium deficiency is a bone disorder. The shape of your body will start to change. You'll lose your posture and you'll have deficiency in your brain and your teeth will develop discoloration. Calcium deficiency causes depression, anxiety, sleep problems, leg pains, cramps, back pain, brittle nails, involuntary twitching, and tingling in your toes and fingers. You can develop joint pain and blood clotting within your body. You'll have problems losing weights, you'll have a loss of strength, be fatigued and can develop heart problems.

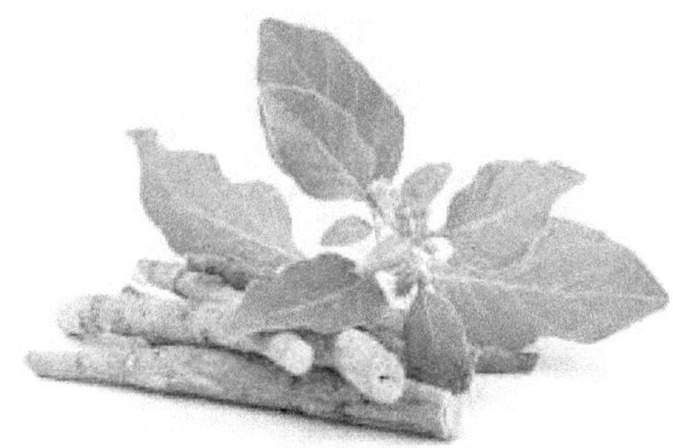

Ashwaganhda

Ashwaganhda fights cough, colds, the flu, and viruses. It gives you strength and energy. It over hauls your body and is great for your nails, hair and your skin. It's great to take to help with your scalp circulation, your thyroids, your brain, and it increases fertility.

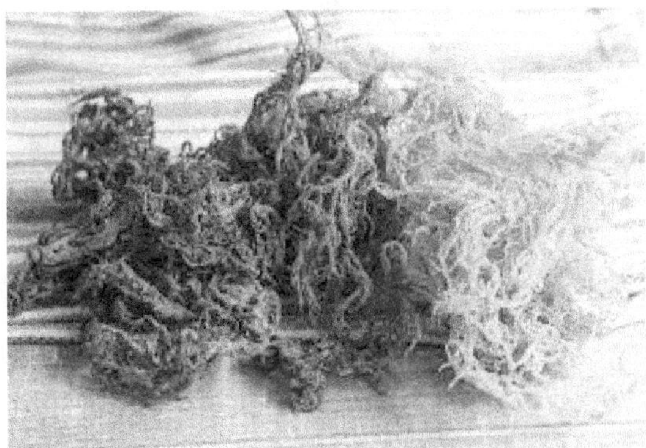

Sea Moss is great if you are diabetic. It's great for colds, mucus, your hair and your bones. It helps to fight radiation poisoning, is good to take if you are going through chemo because it actually helps to fight cancer. It is great for weight loss, it helps to get rid of varicose veins and are great for your arteries. Take sea moss for your skin, teeth and your blood. It's good for the treatment of gout, it's healthy for your heart, your respiratory system, and your sex drive. Sea moss is great for thyroid health. It's an antioxidant and antiviral and it's also good for your immune system and digestive health.

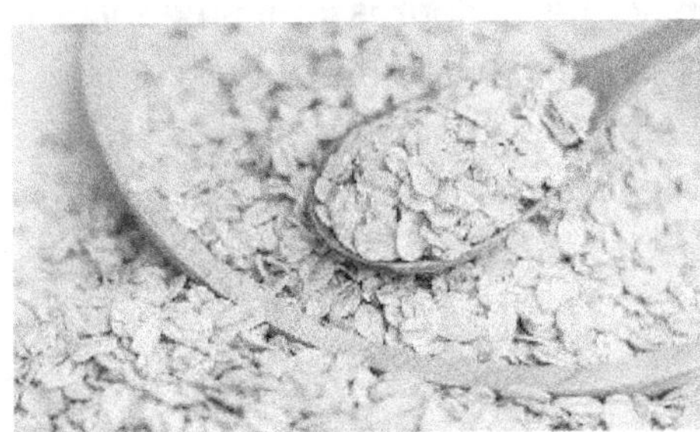

Oatmeal boosts the immune system. It has protein and it reduces asthma in children. Oh, wow, who would have thought that oatmeal can do that? Oatmeal is good for weight loss. It has more antioxidant than broccoli. It helps to prevent cancer and is good for your skin and also helps with longevity.

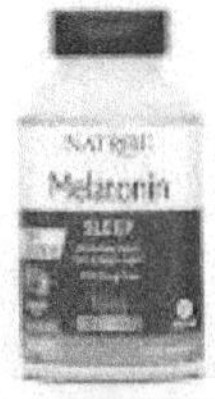

Melatonin helps with sleep, your memory, menopause, jet lag and Alzheimer. It is good to fight off migraines. It helps with your bones and helps to prevent joint pain. Melatonin is great for your heart. It helps with under active fibroid and slows down the aging process. It fights cancer, reduces stress and regulates your blood pressure. You can find Melatonin in pineapples, tart cherries, oatmeal and nuts.

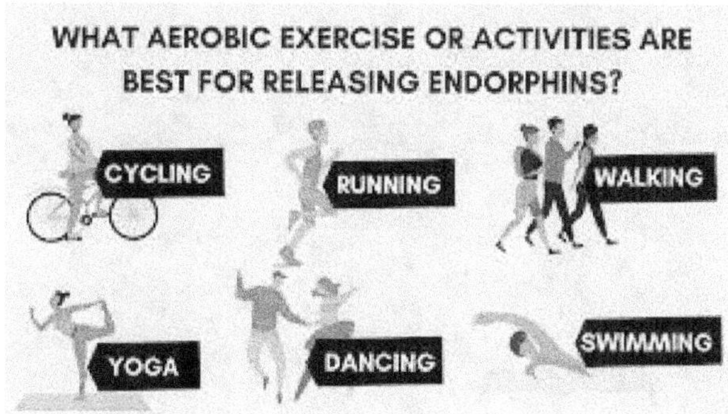

Endorphins

Endorphins are hormones that are already in your body. It relieve pain, stress and the feeling of euphoria. It has the ability to block discomfort. Did you know that it's considered a willpower hormone? It enhances your self-esteem, it gives you positive feelings of confidence, a sense of assurance and a sense of appreciation.

Endorphin deficiencies are chronic pains in the back and neck and chronic headaches. You will become emotionally and physically drained. You'll develop loss of sleep, have a very low pain threshold and you'll be sensitive to bright light. You'll also tear up easily, have cravings for sweets and you won't be able to have fun and can become depressed.

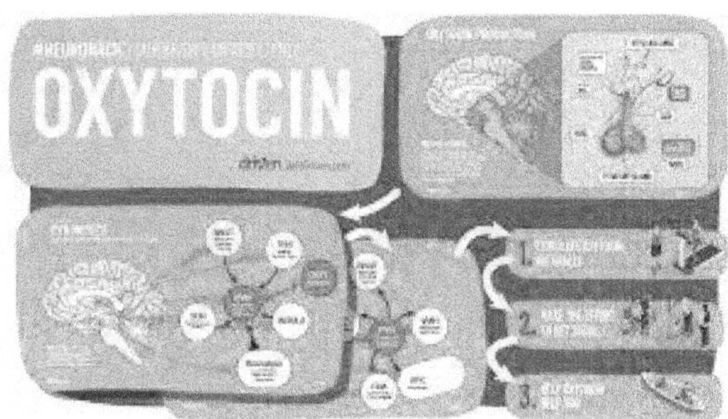

Oxytocin

Oxytocin is already in our bodies. It gives you a feeling of trust and love. It increases your feeling of self-worth, passion, compassion, forgiveness, generosity, joy and security. Oxytocin is received from socializing, acupuncture, music, exercise and deep breathing and also by taking a cold shower, meditation and essential oils. Oxytocin deficiency is a feeling of loneliness, stress, anger, anxiety and insomnia. You'll lack motivation and have sweaty hands, acid reflux and have problems with your bowels.

You can get Oxytocin from figs, avocado, watermelon, spinach, nuts, yogurt, magnesium and probiotics.

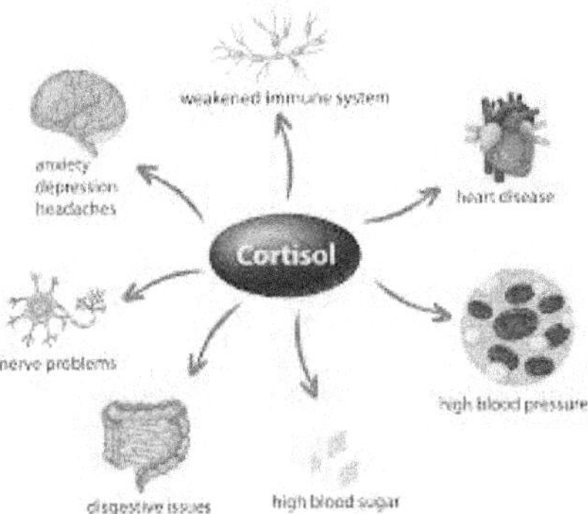

<u>Cortisol</u>

Cortisol is already in our body, it's natures built in alarm system. It helps to maintain your blood pressure and blood sugar. It controls your fear and your moods. It's great for your body and gives you motivation. You want to keep your cortisol low and you can do this by dancing, laughing and by avoiding caffeine and alcohol. Getting a foot massage also helps and so does massage therapy. Watching comedy and being affectionate helps to keep your cortisol in check as well. A high level of cortisol comes from illnesses, surgery, birth control pills, liver or kidney dysfunction, depression and hyper-thyroids.

The symptoms of high cortisol are thinning of the skin, a lack of energy, extreme fatigue, dizziness, sugar and salt cravings, stomachaches in the morning, and a decrease in your immune system. It can cause you to always be sweaty and can cause you to easily bruise. You'll feel flushed, have weight gain and have unusual fat build up. To regulate cortisol, eat garlic, berries, oranges, wild salmon, holy basil, pink Himalaya salt, magnesium, vitamin C, zinc and incorporate foot baths.

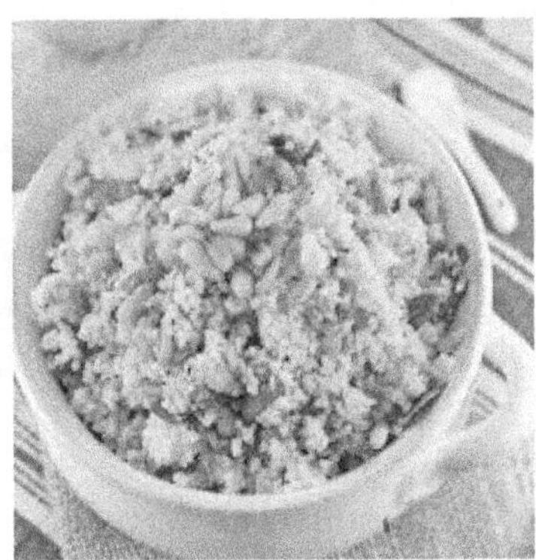

<u>Couscous</u>

Couscous, it sounds funny right? But couscous is sugar free and reduces the risk of prostate and lung cancer. It's cholesterol free and it helps to prevent strokes and heart attacks. Couscous aids in healing wounds faster and improves your muscle mass. It helps with your digestion and and prevent constipation. It kills bacteria, balances the fluid in your body and is great to eat to assist in weight loss. It helps to give you energy and is good for your bones and helps to prevent gout. It's very beneficial for your brain. It increases your memory so it's really great for those suffering with Alzheimer. It helps you to concentrate more and it does wonder for your nervous system. Couscous actually boosts your immune system and prevents depression. It has vitamins B6, B1, B3, iron potassium and vitamin C. It helps to prevent hair loss and can actually lift your mood. If you're going through menopause add this to your diet. It fights colds and the flu. If you or someone you know has type 2 diabetes place this on your menu and it also reduces the risk of bone cancer.

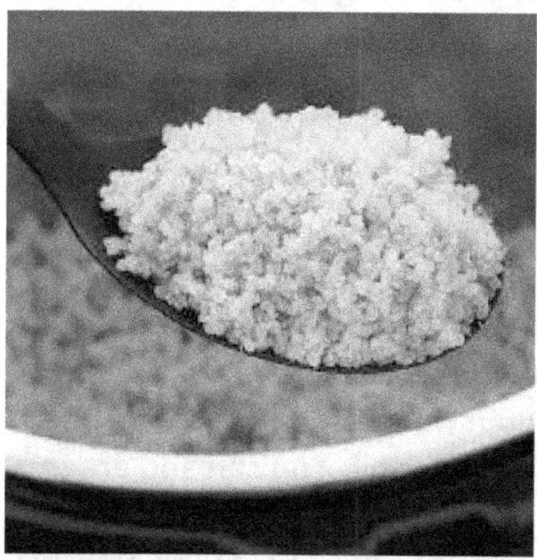
Quinoa

Quinoa is good for bone health, your brain and your mind. It decreases depression and is a great additive to add to someone's diet if the have Alzheimer or Dementia. Quinoa helps with your bowels, reduces migraines, and helps to prevent gallstones. It's good for your heart health and it lowers and balances out your blood pressure. It treats diabetes, prevents breast cancer, and makes a great rice substitute. Can you believe that it's also good for your skin? It helps to fight stress and it lowers lowers your cholesterol. Quinoa has copper, fiber, iron, magnesium, folate, zinc, B9 and potassium. Its good for mental and emotional health and is good for the function of your red cell formation.

Chapter 10
Detoxes

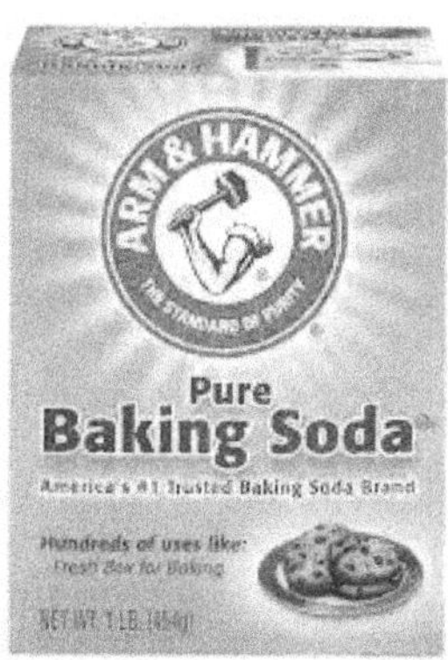
Baking Soda (Detox)

STOP USING TOOTHPASTE USE BAKING SODA INSTEAD! Baking Soda is good for whitening your teeth and it's good for your kidneys. It good to take to fight colds, the flu and viruses. Baking soda is a great for a feet detox bath. It's a cancer prevention, it regulates your blood sugar making it great for Diabetics. It's a good hand cleanser. It helps to eliminate toxins. It fights fungus and helps to clear yellow nails. Baking soda is good for gout and arthritis. It makes a good deodorant and it's good for your digestion. It's great to clean your garbage can, freshens your refrigerator, cleans your toilets and sinks and is a wonderful carpets freshener. It also is good to freshen up your upholstery. Women use baking soda with apple cider vinegar for vaginal discharge.

Detox Bath

A detox bath flushes out toxins and poisons out of your body. It helps to reduce your stress hormones. A detox bath gets rid of rashes, headaches, colds, the flu and viruses. It helps to relive pain and is good for your muscles. You can add essential oil to your bath, such as spearmint, and lavender oil. You can add green tea, ginger, magnesium, milk and honey. You can add clay, sea salt, charcoal, and vanilla oil. Add one cup of Apple Cider Vinegar into your bath to help with arthritis, urinary tract infection, and joint pain.

Raw Vegetable Detox

Raw vegetables give you energy, stamina and mental clarity. They help to keep you emotionally and spiritually balanced. They help to fight diseases and they help you to focus and improves your confidence.Do you know that eating raw vegetables gives you a deeper connection with people, helps to cleanse your organs and is good for your heart.

Detox Teas

Ginger, turmeric, orange peel, rosehip, lemon and lemongrass.

Detox Soups

Kale, collard greens, carrots, broccoli, celery and onion soups are good for detoxing.

Chapter 11

Other Beneficial Things For Your Body

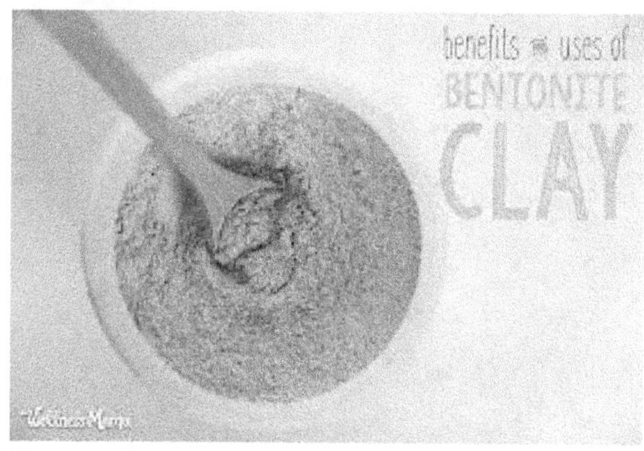

Bentonite

Bentonite strengthens the immune system. Bentonite pulls poisons from your skin and it absorbs moisture. You can use it as a deodorant and a foot detox. It helps with bloating, gas and constipation. You can use it for your scalp and it's good for natural hair, it can actually help your hair to grow. You can put it in your shampoo and sprinkle it on your toothpaste to mineralizes your teeth. It dissolves fat, helps helps if you have food poisoning. It's good for cuts and scars. It improves the oxygen in your body and it alkaline your body. It relieves toxins in your kidneys and your glands. You can add it with Apple Cider Vinegar, cinnamon, cayenne pepper, and lemon to make your lemonade cleanse.

You should detox your kidneys often because if your don't, you will have a difficult and painful urine and your urine will be foamy. The following are good for detoxing your liver, lemon, lime, parsley, dandelion, ginger, turmeric, cabbage, garlic, apple cider vinegar, grapes, carrots, spirulina, blueberries, strawberries, blackberries, cranberries, celery, oregano and Aloe Vera juice.

A Cold Shower

A cold shower helps to boost the immune system. It helps to fight the flu, colds, and coughs. It helps to build up your white blood cells and lowers your blood pressure. It's great for your skin, your arteries, your veins and your blood vessels. A cold shower can actually help your nervous system. It's good for your muscles, it reduces inflammation and swelling and relives muscle soreness, gout, and arthritis.

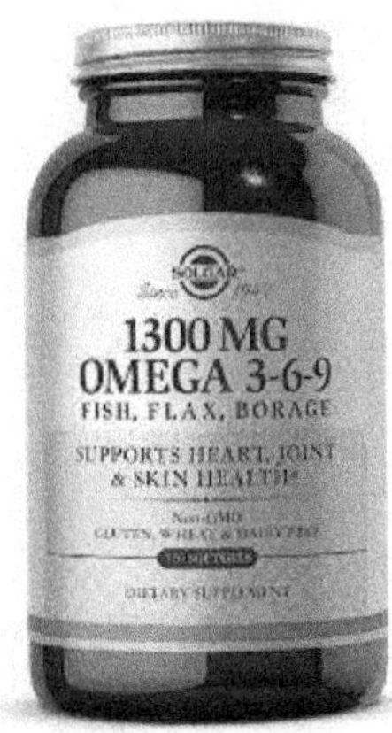

<u>Omega- 3,6,9;</u>

Taking Omega-3,6,9, boosts your immune system. It's great to take for a sore throat, skin, eyes, and helps your brain to function well. They support your nervous system and prevents inflammation and learning disabilities. They also help with your blood circulation. You can get Omega-3,6,9, by eating salmon, tuna, sardines, kale, walnuts, eggs, flax seeds, and chia seeds. They also have iron in it. They are great for arthritis, diabetics, allergies, menopause and your reproductive system. Omega- 3,6,9 is good to take if you have high blood pressure. It's great for hair growth and it helps to fight cancer. You can get Omega 3,6,9 in pill form and powder powder form as well.

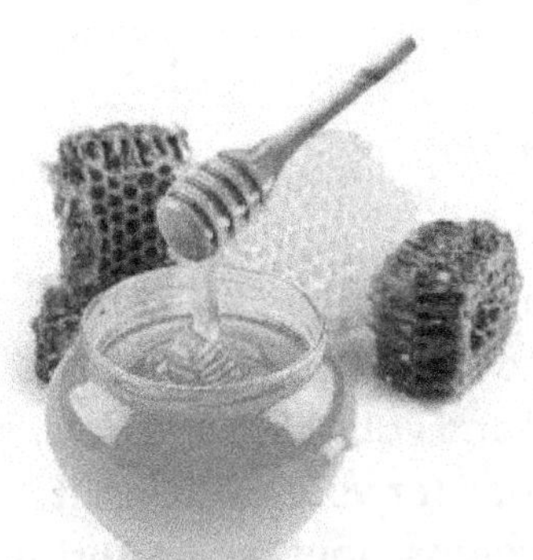

<u>Honey (Raw Honey And Local Honey Is Best)</u>

Honey is not good for babies to consume. Honey fights bacteria, viruses, colds, cough, sore throat and wounds. It's good for your skin, hair and your brain. It gives you energy and helps with your digestion. It has vitamins B3, B5, B2, zinc, vitamin C, magnesium and iron. Honey has twenty-seven minerals.

There are different types of fasting. There's the Water Fast, the Daniel Fast, Juice Fast, and Smoothie Fast and fasting to lose weight. When you fast you, you should be praying, reading and studying the Word of God. You are one on one with the Lord, He should be your main focus. You should be shutting yourself out from those around you.

Fasting boosts the immune system. It regenerates the immune cells, enhances the liver functions and detoxifies the body. Whenever you fast, it helps to heals your body. It's good for your kidneys and it helps you with weight loss. Fasting is good for your digestion, it reduces joint pains and and helps with arthritis. It helps you to stop food craving and it's a good way to start a new eating habit. It lowers your blood sugar making it great for diabetics. It lowers your cholesterol levels, reduces heart problems and can reduce allergies. It also helps you to sleep better. Fasting is good for your skin, mental clarity and your memory. It helps you to focus and within three days it helps to break addictions. Fasting brings you peace and calm in your life. Its great for your liver and it shrinks your stomach. It strengthens you mentally and builds you up. It helps in giving you wisdom and it gives you revelation.

Fasting causes the flesh to decrease spiritually. It gives you a power surge and also builds up your spirit, soul, and body.

Some of the side effects of fasting are dizziness, headaches and a low grade fever. You may experience diarrhea or have symptoms of the flu. This lets you know that your body is removing the toxins out of it and is cleansing itself.

Of course when you fast don't eat fast foods, starches (rice, potatoes, pasta), ice-cream, chips, cake, ice tea, sugary drinks, breads, or junk food.

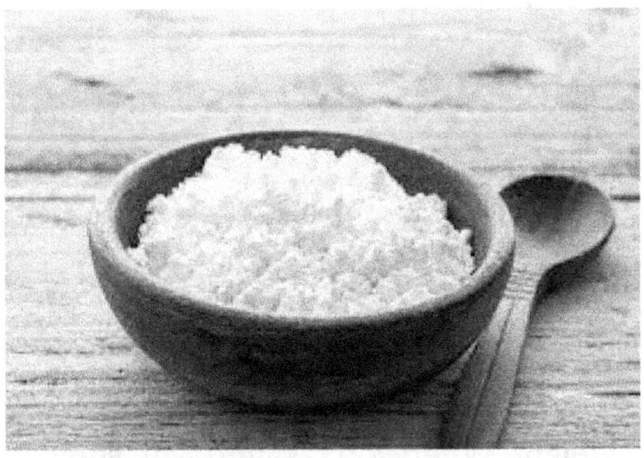

Cottage cheese can help you lose weight. It decreases your level of anxiety and stress. Cottage cheese is good for your bones, arthritis, gout, and your teeth. It helps with muscle cramps and it lowers your blood pressure. It reduces the risk of breast cancer and heart disease. Cottage cheese helps to regulate blood sugar so it's good for diabetics. It boosts the immune system so it's good for colds, coughs, the flu and viruses. It has vitamins B12, D, A, zinc, potassium and calcium. It can help with your thoughts, wow, imagine that! It helps you to feel well and upbeat. It aids with your digestive system, gives you energy and is an anti-aging food.

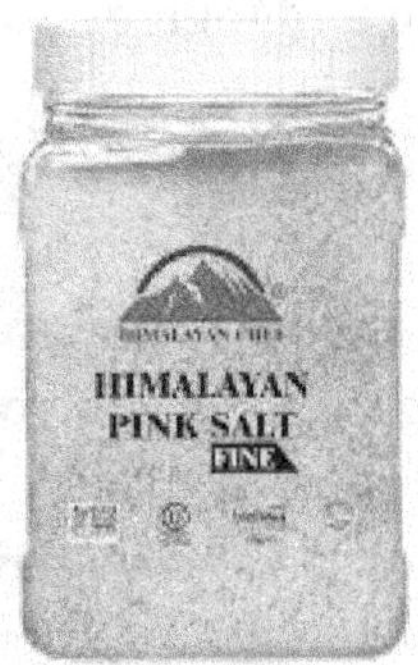

Pink Himalayan Salt

If you're going to use salt, use Pink Himalayan salt because it's a much more healthier salt to use. It has magnesium and calcium. It lowers your blood pressure, helps with your blood flow and helps you to sleep. Can you believe that a spice can do all of that? Yes, it, can!

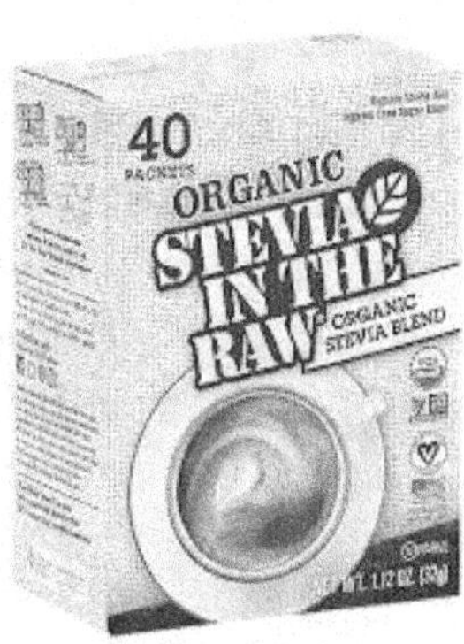 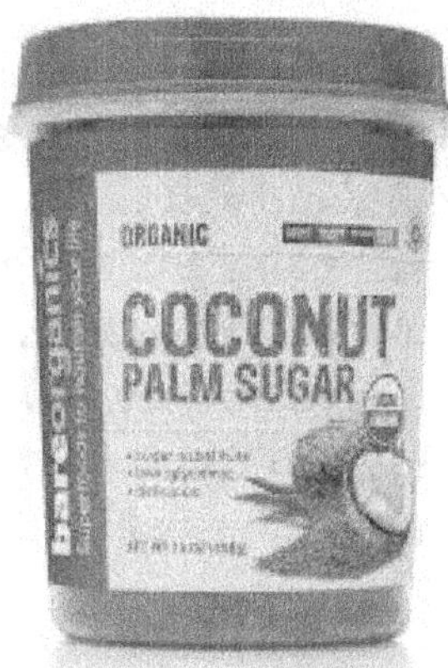

White Sugar is not good for you because it can cause your blood pressure to go up. It gives you a higher risk of developing cancer and it increases the risk of heart disease and strokes. White sugar causes tooth decay, bloating and can give you a fatty liver. It causes your energy to drain, it impairs your memory and is bad for your skin. Use Stevia or Coconut Palm sugar instead.

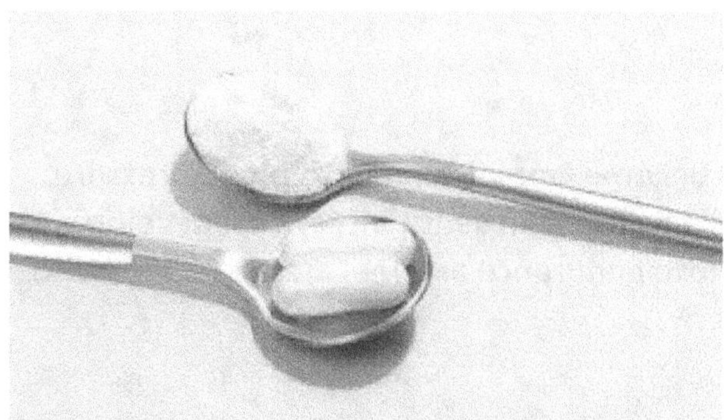

Collagen

Collagen is good for your joints, bones, hair, muscle, skin and nails. It strengthens your brain and is good for gut health. It helps to prevent sagging skin and a sagging butt, uh oh. It also helps to get rid of cellulite and it has vitamin C.

Chapter 12
Deficiencies

Vitamin B6

Vitamin B6 deficiency affects your mental health and your physical health. You'll become depressed and overwhelmed a lot. You can have feelings of rejection and have mood swings. You can develop feelings of inadequacy. You can become anemic and develop cracks in your mouth. You'll have chapped lips and a sore and swollen tongue. Your skin will have dry patches and you can develop heart problems. You can have problems with your eyes and always be tired. You'll have a loss of appetite and loss of taste. You can actually develop seizures. Vitamin B6 helps to prevent cancer and helps to cure the covid-19.

Iron Deficiency

Iron deficiency can cause you to become anemic and it can impair your immune system. Your can develop an irregular heart beat and your tongue will get discolored. You'll have dry mouth and you will have frequent infections such as yeast infections. You'll have chest pains and will become weak and fatigued. You won't be able to concentrate or focus. You can develop memory loss. You'll have cold hands and cold feet. You'll have anxiety, dry skin and your skin will become yellow. Your hair will dry out and you'll become dizzy and light headed. It will also make you have a poor appetite and unusual food cravings. Eating ice is a sign of iron deficiency.

B12 Deficiency And Lack Of The B Complex

The lack of the B complex and B12 can cause brain damage, rapid heart beat and makes your thinking slow. It makes you weary and depressed. The lack of B12 can cause infertility and will keep you from being motivated. It gives you a loss of appetite and gives you shortness of breath. You can actually become diabetic. You'll have problems with your bowels, develop mouth ulcers and canker sores.

Vitamin D Deficiency

The lack of vitamin D can cause you to become cranky, have high blood pressure, develop muscle weakness and you will develop pain sensitivity. You'll develop bone fractures and bone aches. You'll lose endurance and feel drained. You'll also have brain fog and will always feel sleepy.

Folate

The lack of Folic comes from poor eating habits, alcohol, GI tract, junk food, some medication and pregnancy. The lack of folate causes fatigue, weakness, exhaustion, mouth sores, headaches and an irregular heart rhythm. The lack of folate causes a swollen tongue, shortness of breath and cracks in the corner of your mouth. You can become very irritable. You will have a decline in your brain function and you won't be able to concentrate and you can be confused. You may have a loss of appetite, develop numbness, have unusual weight loss and get depressed. You'll have a feeling of despair and it can causes birth defects. You'll have diarrhea and it could stunt growth. You can have premature gray hair and problems with your digestive system.

Chapter 13

Essential Oils

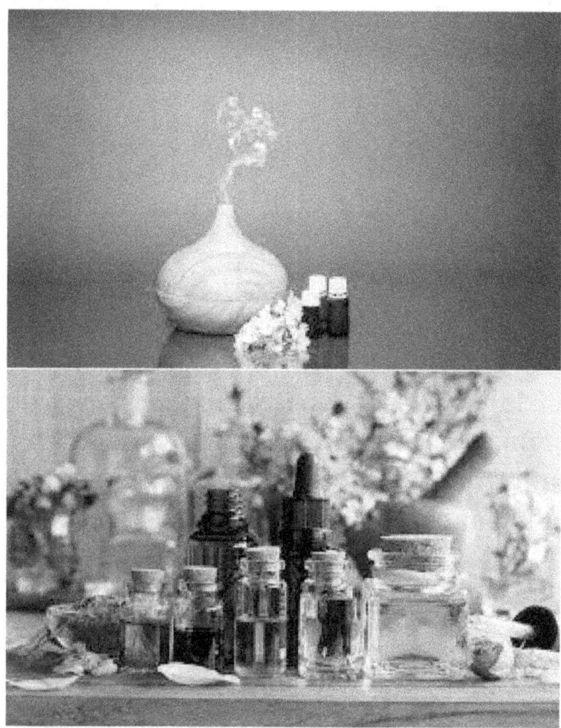

Essential Oils Are Wonderful. And believe it or not they can boost the immune system. They give you a peace of mind and they smell great. They also have many benefits. You can mix your own oils together and create your own smells. When you purchase essential oils make sure that they are 100% pure. There are some essential oils that you can put under your tongue to get the full benefits. You need to put essential oils into a diffuser, there are so many different types to choose from. Essential oils are good to rub on your skin but make sure to dilute it with a carrier oil because the oils dissolve into your skin. You can use coconut oil, olive oil, jojoba oil, avocado oil, and castor oil to use as a carrier oil just to name a few. There are some oils that you can actually use on your skin such as coconut, and olive oil. Some people's skin may be more sensitive than others so make sure to do a skin test before putting anything on your skin, especially if you have never used essential oils before. There are oils that you can open and inhale to get instant relief such as eucalyptus and lavender oil, these are just a few. Once you open a bottle, you'll be able to smell for yourself to see what effects you may have. There are essential oils that detoxes the body, and they are, oregano, lemongrass, lemon and avocado. They have vitamins B, C, and K and they give you energy, and are good for the heart.

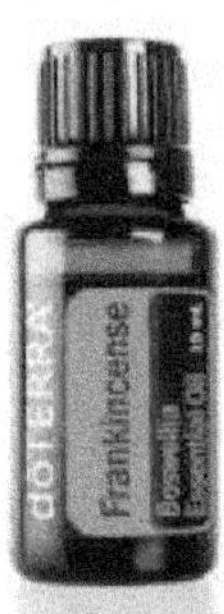

Frankincense 100%

Frankincense Oil was once worth more than gold. It helps with your mood because it's an antidepressant and it helps with anxiety and sadness. It's good for back pain, your feet, skin, nails and stretch marks. Frankincense is good for cyst, warts, wrinkles and scars. It helps promote urination and is good for your digestion. Many essential oils you can digest and if you use them on your skin use a carrier oil along with it.

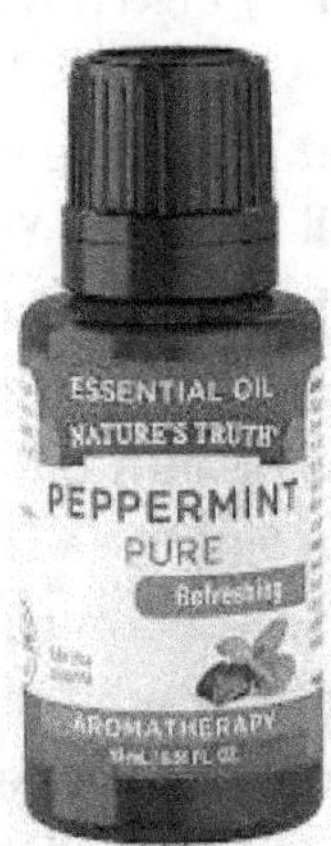

Peppermint 100%

Peppermint oil is good for massages. It's good for your stomach, it helps with your mood and helps to relive muscle pain. It's good for your if you're running a fever, have a cold, a cough, the flu or a virus. It helps to treat herpes! It's good for your neck, hands, knees and your skin. Peppermint oil is good for your colon, teeth and your gums. You can rub it on your temple if you have a headache. It's good for your hair and nails. It helps you to relax and focus, and it helps you to concentrate and to keep you alert. It helps with bloating, arthritis, and your respiratory tract. Peppermint oil helps with breast cancer, diarrhea and tumors. It also helps to fight bacteria.

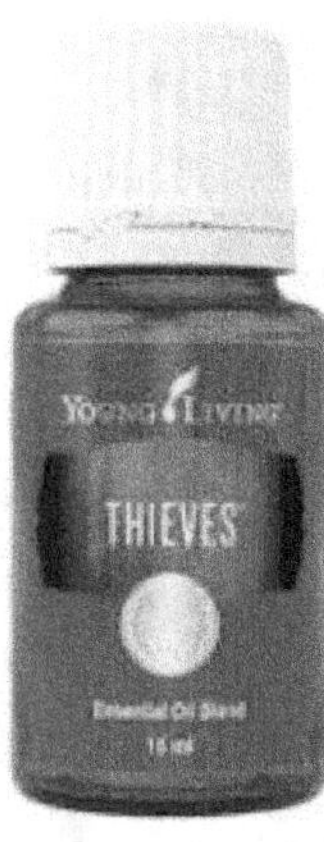

Thieves Oil 100%

Thieves oil helps to fight infections and you can actually gargle with it. It helps to give you longevity, oh my goodness, that's great! It's good for acne, It fights colds and the flu. It protects your immune system by fighting viruses. It gets rid of germs and helps to fight gum disease and cavities. It gets rid of phlegm, mold, tumors and staph disease. It helps your kidneys and liver and it's good for diabetics. It's soothing, uplifting and energizing.

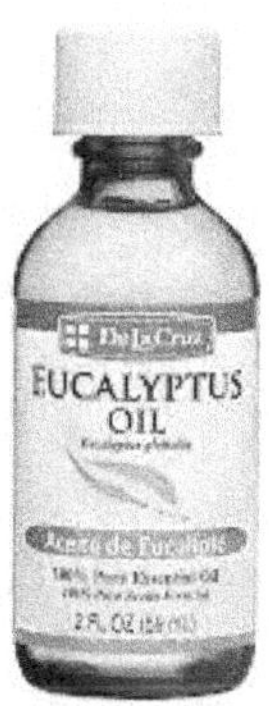

Eucalyptus Oil 100%

Eucalyptus oil is good if you are congested because it aids with your breathing. It's good for inflammation, viruses and the covid-19 virus as well. It helps to fight colds, and the flu. Use eucalyptus oil for the shingles, burns, allergies and pneumonia. Eucalyptus oil helps with your sinuses and fights stress and insomnia. Put eucalyptus oil in a diffuser to help with your mental state. It is good to have this in a sickroom, just inhale the fumes. It's good for your skin, wounds and cuts but make sure to use a carrier oil to help to dilute it if you're going to put it on your skin. It's also good to rub on you if you have arthritis.

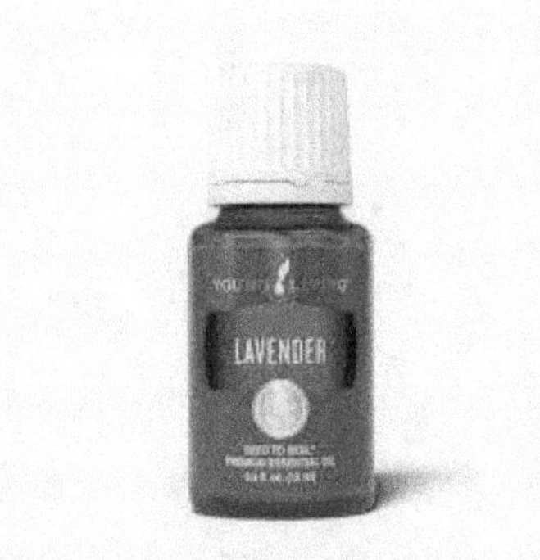

<u>Lavender Oil 100%</u>

Lavender can be used as perfume. It clears the air, helps with hair growth and is good to help you sleep because it's so calming. It's good for migraines, stress and anxiety. Lavender oil helps to fight wrinkles, acne, helps to remove dark spots and soothes sore feet. It's good for your respiratory system and your intestines. Lavender oil is good for your digestion and your nerves. It can also help to get rid of fungus. It boosts your immune system so it helps to fight the flu, colds, cough, and viruses. It's good for diabetics. You can use it as a deodorant and you can put it into the wash to make the laundry smell fresh. It's good for your nerves because the smell relaxes you.

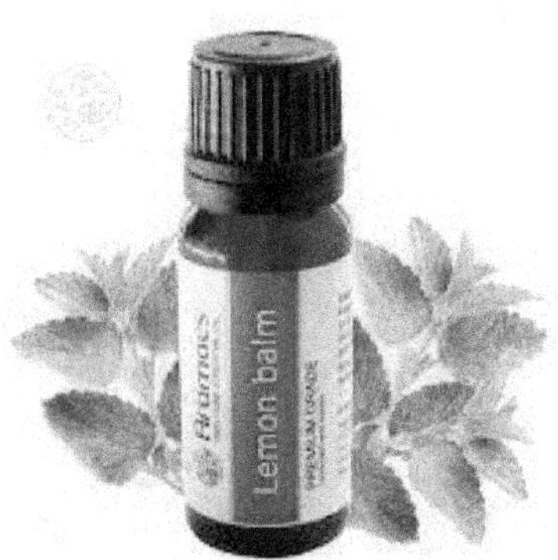

<u>Lemon Balm Oil 100%</u>

Lemon balm oil lowers your blood pressure and is good for your brain. It helps you to concentrate, stay focused and alert. It helps you to be enthusiastic and is good to help to rid of staph and cold sores. It reduces bloating, helps with insomnia and gas. It helps to relive headaches. Use lemon balm oil for colds, cough, the flu, and viruses. It boosts the immune system and is good to fight off covid-19. Lemon balm dispels nightmares, depression, and its a calming oil. It helps to fight heartburn and is good for your heart and liver. It helps if you have acid reflux. It helps your colon, arthritis and gout. You can put lemon balm in lotions and deodorant. It helps to get rid a toothache, it fight cancer cells and bacteria, it's also good for allergies.

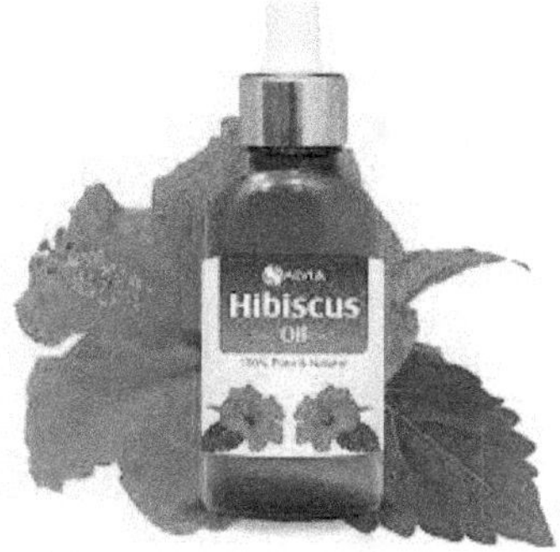

Hibiscus Oil 100%

Hibiscus oil is good for you if you have high blood pressure but it's not good if you have low blood pressure. It helps to lower your cholesterol and is good to fight colds, cough, the flu and viruses. It fights bacteria and staph and is good for depression, stress and anxiety. Looking to lose weight? Get this oil, it can help with your weight loss journey. Hibiscus oil is great for your heart and liver. It slows aging and it helps with constipation and insomnia. It's good for your urinary tract and it helps to fight infections. It has vitamins A, K, zinc, and has the B complex.

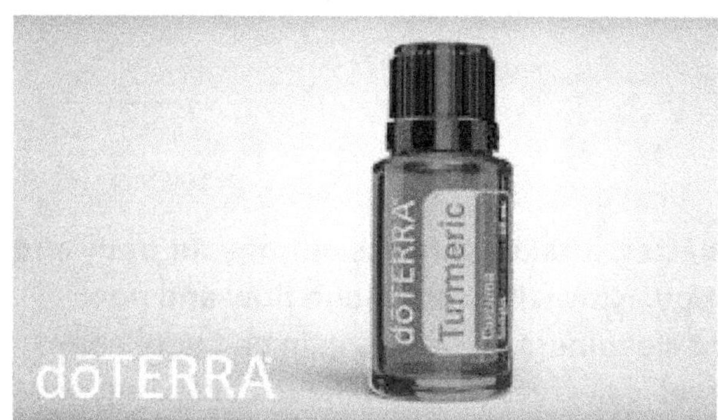

Tumeric Oil 100%

Turmeric oil is good for your skin, nails, lips, scars. It's help to get rid of spots on your skin. It's good for the soles of your feet, your brain. Tumeric oil fights joint pains and back pains. It's good for you knees and helps to fight seizures. It helps to fight viral infections and the flu. This oil is good in fighting leukemia and helps with your mood swings. Tumeric oil is great if you or someone you know has dementia because it's great for your brain and can increase your memory. It gives you positive thoughts and helps to clear cloudy thinking. Tumeric oil is a wonderful oil to use to balance your emotions. It helps with hopelessness, fear and despair. It helps you to sleep well, it gives you energy and helps to boost your immune system.

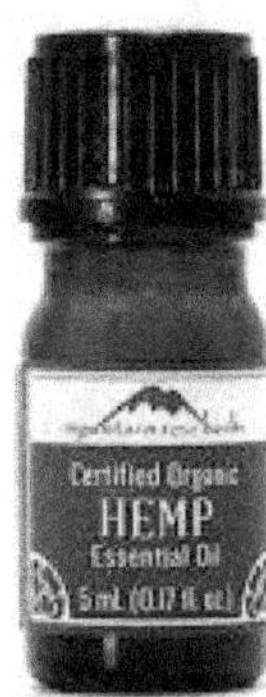

<u>Hemp Oil 100%</u>

Hemp oil fights bacteria growth and regulates your blood sugar making it good for you if you're diabetic. It helps to prevent convulsions and it helps to prevent vomiting. It helps to fight seizures, muscle cramps, fear, depression, anxiety and mental illness. It helps the nervous system and it helps you to rest. Hemp oil helps to fight cancer, inflammation and pain. It helps to build body tissue and is good for your heart, small intestines and your organs. It has protein and amino acids and it also boosts your immune system.

<u>Chapter 14</u>

Last But Not Least Things

<u>Signs Of Poor Circulation and Poor Blood Flow</u>

A good blood flow helps you to think better, it takes stiffness out of your body and makes you more positive and more happy. Now with poor blood flow and poor blood circulation you will have constant sleepiness, excessive gain and you'll have a poor immune system. Your energy level is decreased, you'll have cold hands, feet, ears, and nose. You'll get dizzy after changing your sitting position. You'll have difficulty reading and your attention span will be decreased. You'll have a slow healing process, have deep skin wrinkles and dry skin. You'll have numbness and tingling in your feet and legs. You'll have memory fog and a lack of focus.

Things that are good to help your blood to flow well are, coconut oil, avocado, watermelon, sunflower seeds, herbal tea, vitamin C and B3. Drink plenty of water. Did you know that your body rebuilds itself in two years? When you rest and sleep your body repairs itself, 98% of your body is always regenerating itself. The cells in your body eventually die and are replaced by new cells. This can happen by eating well by eating the right foods and drinking the right things and also, don't forget to exercise. Every morning your brain cells renews itself. Your DNA renews itself every two months. Your skin rebuilds itself in one month. Your liver rebuilds itself in six weeks. Your stomach lining rebuilds itself in five days. Your brain rebuilds itself in one year. Your blood rebuilds itself in four months and your bone rebuilds itself in three months. Our bodies are absolutely amazing that's why we have to eat the right things to keep it going and help it to heal itself.

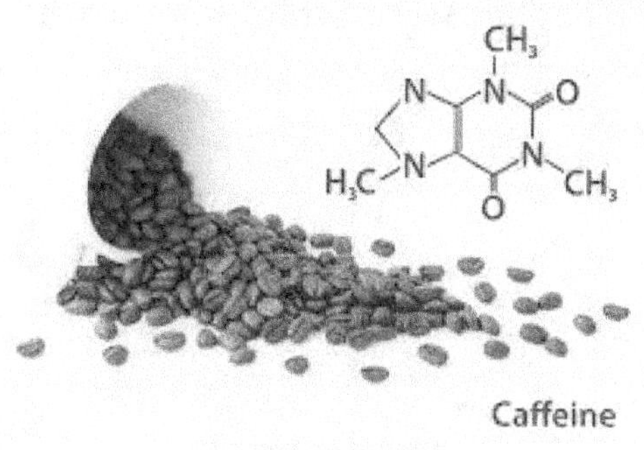

Caffeine

Caffeine is not good for your body and is found in candy that is why children are bouncing off of the walls when they eat too much of it. It's also found in medicine and desserts. Caffeine causes headaches and increases urination and diarrhea. You'll have rapid heart beat, muscle aches, painful breasts and lumps in the breasts. Your bones will deteriorate and you'll have an increase in your blood pressure. You'll have heartburn and be irritable. Caffeine withdrawal causes brain fog, brain pain and drowsiness. You will become moody and have flu-like symptoms. Overall caffeine is not very good for you.

A caffeine overdose causes flashes in your eyes, ringing in the ears and causes trembling and twitching. You can have seizures and kidney problems. You can become restless and confused. You may also have insomnia and an irregular heart beat.

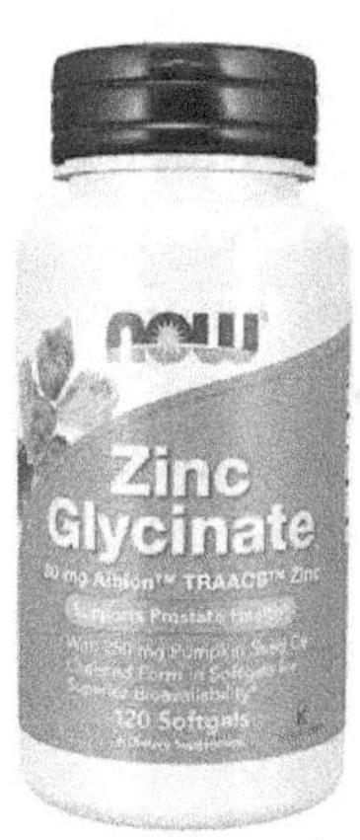

Zinc

Zinc strengthens your bones, helps to fight arthritis and enhances the cells in your body. Zinc builds up your immune system and reduces the need of antibiotics. It helps in weight loss and improves your sense of smell and vision. It also helps to regulate your body. It helps with your memory, regulates your blood sugar and helps with fertility by increasing the sperm count. So if you're trying to have a baby, tell your husband to start taking zinc. Zinc fights chronic fungus infection and maintains a strong brain function. Zinc is great for Alzheimer and Dementia. Zinc cures bruises and bumps. It causes energy to flow in the brains of babies and is good for pregnancy.

You can find Zinc in carrots, brown rice, lentil, eggs, chicken, spinach, nuts, mushrooms, sesame seeds, most fruits, lamb, Kiefer, yogurt and cocoa.

Zinc deficiency is a loss of smell and taste, low blood pressure, white spots under the nails, pale skin and rough skin.

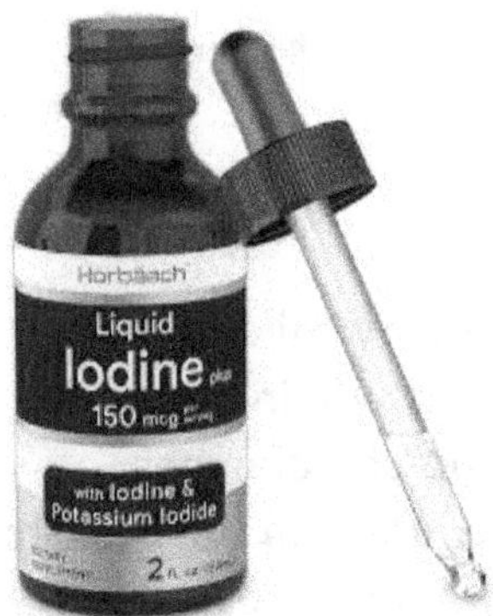

Iodine

Iodine supports your thyroid glands and helps to fight cancer. It's good for your brain health and helps you to recover from radiation. It regulates your hormones and strengthens and builds up your immune system. It maintains a healthy energy level, is good for pregnant women and it helps to fight yeast infections and other infections as well.

Sweating

Sweating protects your heart, cleanses your body and detoxes your body. Sweating helps to regulate the temperature of your body as well. It's good for your blood circulation and is good for your skin, brain and your memory. When you sweat it helps to fight germs and it also helps to prevent kidney stones. Sweating helps to lower your stress hormones and makes you happier. Sweating increases the serotonin in your body and it cleanses your skin. Sweating reduces menopause and andropause plus it relaxes your body and your mind. It improves your sleep, it helps to fight colds, the flu and virus.

Music

Music reduces stress and anxiety. It has the ability to drive out depression and will make you feel well in your spirit, soul and body. The wrong music can actually make you sick. Gospel music will lift your spirit and make you have a feeling of wellness. Music creates creative thinking and enhances your blood vessel function. It releases your serotonin that makes your feel better. It's great for your brain because it stimulates it and it helps to lower your blood pressure. It has the ability to relax you and helps you to eat less, yes eat less! It's good therapy for those who has cancer and has a healing effect, especially the harp. It's wonderful for stroke patients. Music improves your coordination and is great for unborn babies. Music boosts your memory and it lifts your mood. Music helps to improve your reading

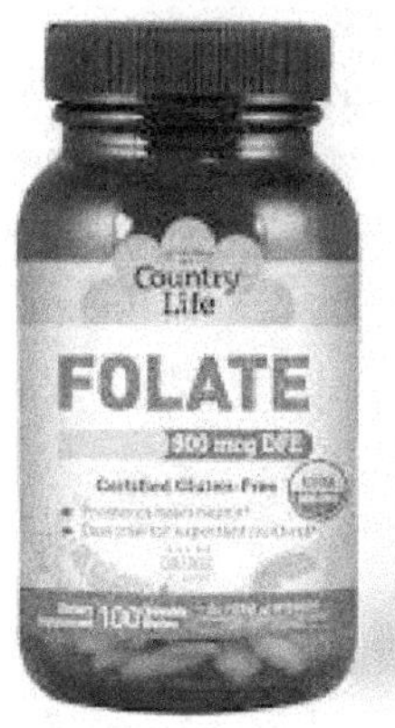

Folate

Folate reduces the risk of strokes and improves the levels of your hemoglobin. It helps with your blood circulation and helps to prevent cancer. Folate reduces the risk of brain defect in babies and the fetus. It assists in a healthy sperm production, repairs skin cells and slows down aging. It gives you energy, promotes growth and helps to maintain muscle and body tissues. Folate promotes healthy brain function and helps to prevent the aging of the brain. Folate is good for your memory, helps with mood disorders and sadness. You can find Folate in brussel sprouts, beans, okra, cauliflower, beets, bell pepper,papaya, broccoli and spinach.

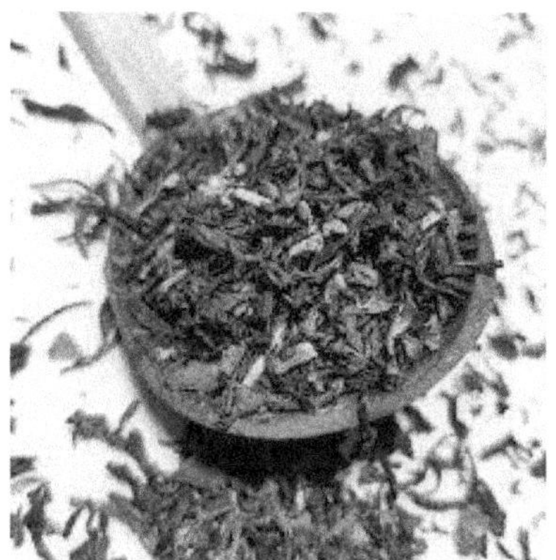

Darjeeling Tea

Darjeeling Tea comes from the mountains of India and are considered the champagne of the teas. It contains low levels of caffeine and has vitamin C which of cause helps with colds, coughs, and the flu. This tea is great for the health of your bones by helping to fight arthritis and gout. It supports your mental activity helping you to concentrate and focus more. Darjeeling tea reduces stress, depression and anxiety. This tea can actually help you to feel good about yourself. It is great for heart health because it fights heart attacks. It fights strokes and strengthens and build up your immune system. Darjeeling tea fights stomach diseases and stomach ailments. It lowers cholesterol and supports your digestion. It increases your energy level and supports dental health.

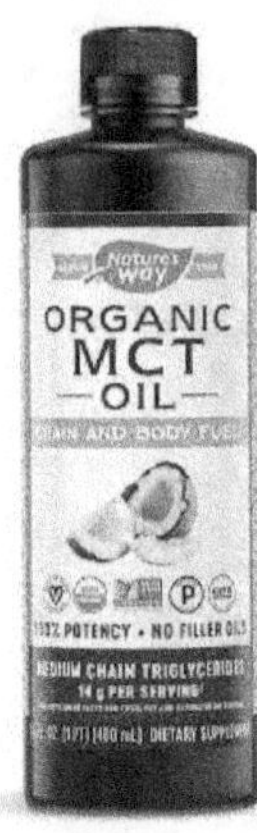

<u>MCT Oil</u>

MCT Oil give your brain power, helping you to focus more and increasing your mentality. It boosts your mood and endurance and helps you to sustain energy. It regulates your appetite and helps you to exercise longer by increasing your stamina. MCT Oil fights inflammation, reduces fatigue, and helps to fight seizures. This oil helps to develop healthy hormones. It's good for your skin and it helps to prevent yeast infections and skin infections as well. This oil is great to give to those is are suffering with autism. It has vitamin C and helps to get rid of thrash. MCT Oil helps to burn fat so if you are on a weight loss journey take some of this oil to help you along the way. MCT Oil also gives your brain power and energy. It increases your endurance for exercise and reduces fatigue and tiredness.

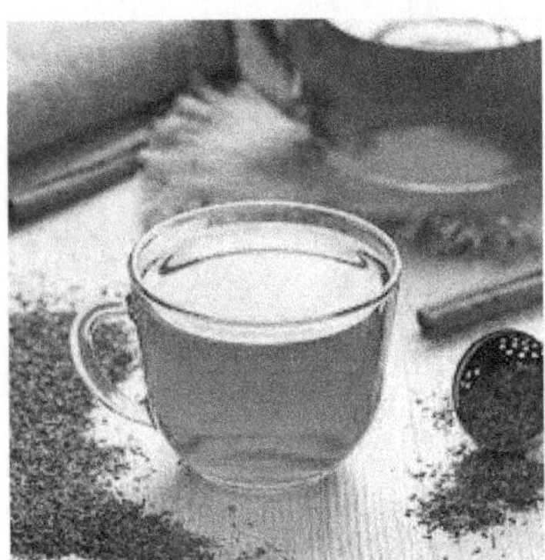

<u>Rooibos Tea</u>

Rooibos Tea is considered a super food. It delays aging, it helps to fight pimples and helps to prevent acne. This tea is great for the function of your brain, it helps you to focus and concentrate more. It increases the airflow to your lungs and reduces tumor growth. You should avoid this tea if you are going through chemo therapy. Rooibos tea contains vitamins C, zinc and calcium. It helps if you have gout or arthritis, it actually helps to reduce the pain. It reduces the risk of heart attacks, it lowers your blood pressure, and reduces muscle soreness. This tea dissolves kidney stones so it extremely good for your kidneys. It helps to prevent diabetes so if you or someone you know suffers with diabetes tell them to add this tea to their diet. Rooibos tea do wonders for a colicky baby. It fights stomach pain and inflammation also.

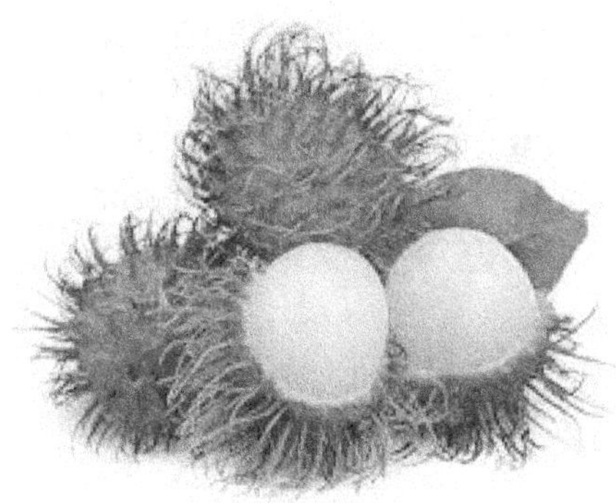

Rambutan Fruit

Rambutan fruit may look like a weird but this fruit boosts your immune system. It had vitamins C, potassium, magnesium, and calcium. Eating this fruit can treat hypertension and builds up your red and white blood cells. It improves sperm count so if you are having problems getting pregnant give your husband some of this fruit to eat. Rambutan fights infections, it regulates your blood sugar and gives you energy. This fruit is great for your kidneys by removing the waste from it. It promotes weight loss and gives you energy.

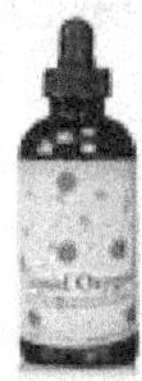

Liquid Oxygen

We all need oxygen, but isn't wonderful to know that you can actually have liquid oxygen? Liquid oxygen can take away headaches but you should always dilute it before taking it. It helps to build new blood vessels, it detoxes your body, and speeds up wounds. It helps to fight heart disease and is good to take of you have asthma. Liquid oxygen promotes nerve growth in the brain and fights cancer. It reduces swelling and is great to take if you are suffering from high blood pressure. Liquid oxygen helps to fight infections in your body, it makes you feel good and it boosts your immune system.

Mindful Breathing

Mindful breathing is just being more conscience on how you are breathing like closing your eyes and inhale through your nose and exhale slowly through your mouth.When you do this you can actually relax yourself and you strengthen lungs. Be aware of the air going up your nostrils. Try to get around fresh air when you are doing your mindful breathing. Get away from cigarette smoke or any smoke of any kind. Take twenty minutes to do mindful breathing. It's best to do this outside, standing in your doorway, or your window and if your going to breath with your window open make sure that your screen is clean Doing this type of breathing relaxes your mind and your body. Doing this type of breathing can lower your blood pressure and it relives emotional distress. This breathing will build up your immune system and it helps to get rid of poisons and toxins in your body. Breathing this way relives your emotions and has the ability to change your mood set. It improves your nervous system. Mindful breathing helps your food to digest well and helps to increase the strength of your muscles. It improves your posture and it strengthens your heart.

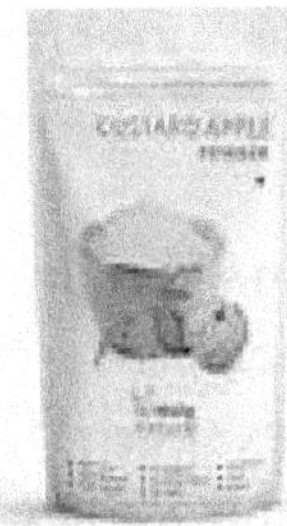

Apple Custard

Apple custard is not intended for pregnant women. It contains vitamins C, B, A, magnesium, and fiber. It helps to fight the cold, coughs, and the flu. It relives stress and can help to keep you from being irritable. It's good to take if you are under weight. It removes fatigue and weakness and it gives you energy. Apple custard helps with your vision and elevates your serotonin. It prevents inflammation and is good for your skin and hair.

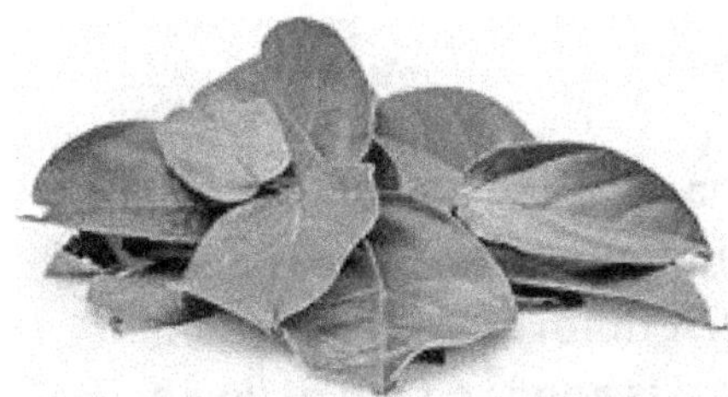

Jelly Grass (Divine Grass)

Jelly Grass leaves contains vitamins A, B C, magnesium, calcium, chlorophyll, chlorella and fiber.It fight against colds, the flu, and coughs. I helps with your bowel movements and constipation. It's good for your digestive system and it cleanses all of your organs. It prevents heartburn and is very useful to assist in your weight loss journey. It reduces the risk of strokes and heart attacks. Jelly Grass kills tumor cells and cancer cell. It kills 55-90% of cancer cells. It helps to prevent breast cancer and cervical cancer as well. Theses leaves are as natural antibiotic. It kills viruses and bacterial. It's great for diabetes, it treats fevers, and eases muscle pains, soreness and muscle stiffness. Jelly Grass is good for your hair, helps dry skin, and is known to cure ulcers.

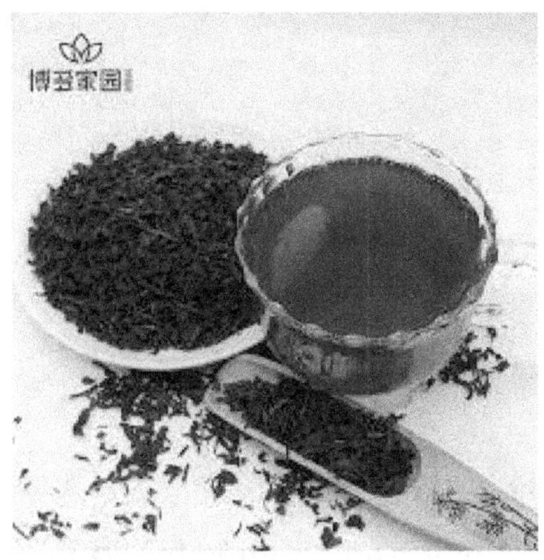

Black Tea

Black Tea strengthens your bones making it very helpful if you suffer with arthritis or gout. It kills bacteria and helps to prevent cancer. It helps you to focus mentally and it lowers depression. Black Tea helps to fight Parkinson Disease, is great to fight memory loss and fights liver disease. If you suffer with asthma have a nice cup of black tea. It fights intestinal disorders and headaches. It lowers the risk of diabetes and helps to get rid of oily skin. It curbs premature aging, aids in the function of your brain and enhances your blood flow and your blood circulation.

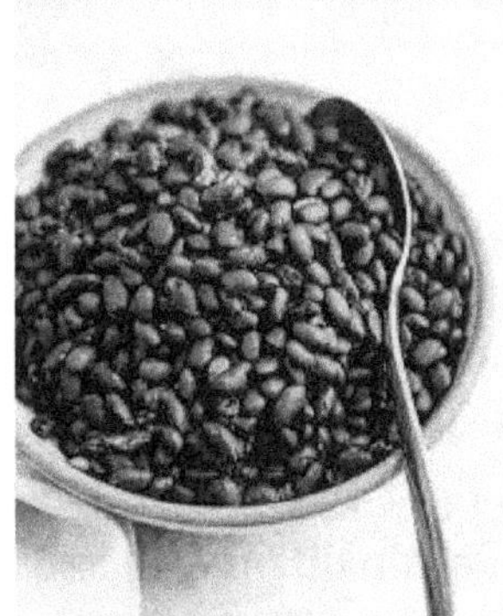

Black Beans

Black beans contains vitamins B1, B6, B3, folate, magnesium, calcium, and iron. It reduces erectile dysfunction in men and reduces the risk of cancer. It also helps to prevent inflammation.

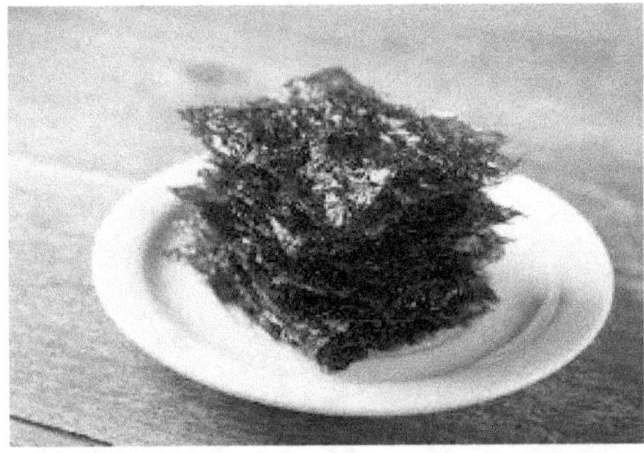

Seaweed supports your bones and tissues. It's rich in iodine and is good for your thyroids. It builds up your blood and iron making it a great addition to your diet if you are anemic. It's great for the health of your heart and it fights diabetes. Seaweed strengthens your nails and helps them to grow. It also conditions your skin.

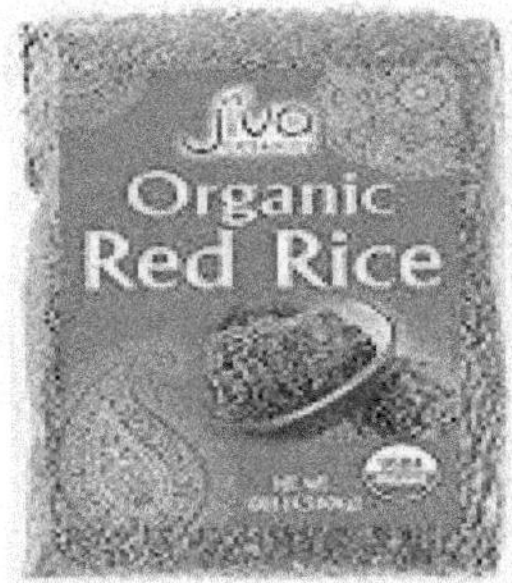

Red Rice (Organic)

Organic red rice is rich in vitamins and minerals such as magnesium, zinc, iron, and fiber. It's great to assist in the health of your bones helping to fight against arthritis and gout. It helps to fight asthma and kidney problems. It's an antioxidant and it boosts your digestive system. It helps with weight loss and it helps to fight fatigue. Organic red rice helps to prevent heart disease and is great for the health of your heart. It helps to fight against arthritis and gout and it lowers your cholesterol.

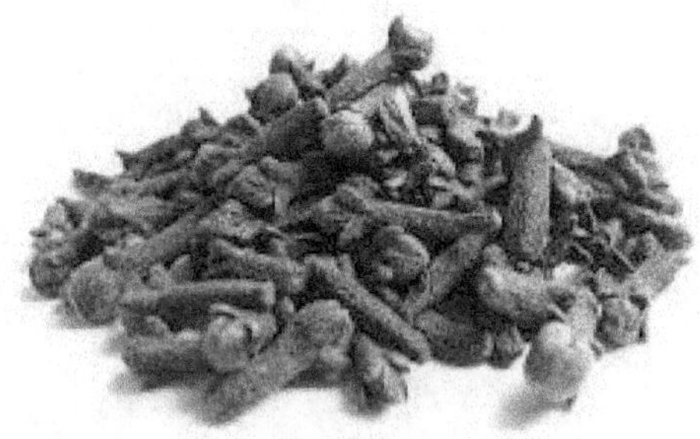

Cloves

Cloves helps to fight respiratory infections and the symptoms of a cold. It helps to relive gas and mouth ulcers. It makes a good mouth wash antiseptic and helps with teeth problems. It fights parasites and helps to keep your lungs and liver healthy.

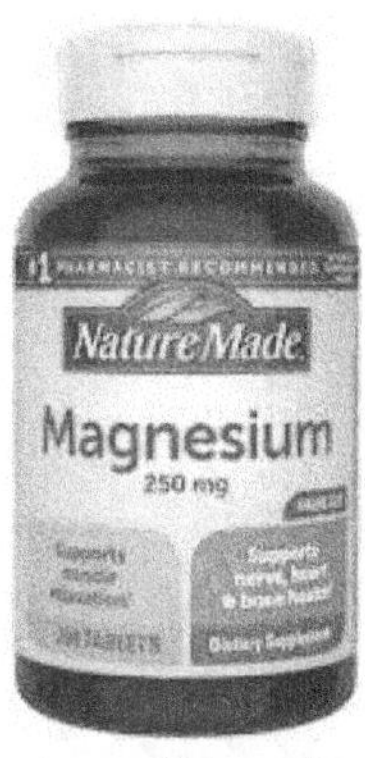

Magnesium (Benefits)

Magnesium protects you against diabetes and reduces high blood pressure. It supports bone health and strengthens bone density. It protects your heart and helps your veins and arteries. It combats asthma and relives insomnia. Magnesium relives constipation and helps you to digest your food. It boosts your energy on a cellular level. It helps your bladder to function well and helps to prevent frequent urination. It improves your mental performance, improves your thinking and gives energy in your mind. Magnesium reduces stress and it helps to absorb the minerals that you take, it also builds and boosts your immune system.

Magnesium deficiency will give you tingling in your fingers and hands. It will cause cramping in the soles of your feet and toes. You will develop cramps in your thighs and calf. You'll have feelings of weakness and it can cause you to have kidney stones and brittle bones.